BEE VENOM

THE NATURAL CURATIVE
FOR ARTHRITIS AND RHEUMATISM

Bee Venom

THE NATURAL CURATIVE FOR ARTHRITIS
AND RHEUMATISM

New Foreword by Harold Goodman, D.O.

Joseph Broadman, M.D.

HEALTH RESOURCES PRESS, INC.

Health Resources Press, Inc.
8609 Second Ave., Suite 405-B
Silver Spring, Maryland 20910

Telephone: 301-565-2494
Website: www.drharoldgoodman.com

New and used books on alternative medicine

THIS BOOK IS INTENDED TO INTRODUCE THE READER TO ALTERNATIVE APPROACHES TO TREATMENTS FOR DISEASE, AND TO BETTER UNDERSTAND ALTERNATIVE ASPECTS OF THERAPY. ITS INTENT IS EDUCATIONAL. THIS BOOK SHOULD NOT BE SUBSTITUTED FOR THE ADVICE AND TREATMENT OF A LICENSED PHYSICIAN. THE AUTHOR AND PUBLISHER DISCLAIM RESPONSIBILITY FOR ANY ADVDERSE EFFECTS RESULTING FROM THE INFORMATION CONTAINED HEREIN.

ISBN 9781890708016

Printed and bound in the United States of America.

The paper used in this publication meets the minimum requirements of American National Standard for Information Sciences - Permanence of Paper for Printed Library Materials, ANSI Z39.48-1984.

TO MY LATE BROTHER

NATHANIEL BROADMAN, M.D.

whose scientific curiosity led to my interest in the treatment of rheumatic diseases, this volume is dedicated.

FOREWORD TO 1997 EDITION

When the history of bee venom therapy is finally written, the name of Joseph Broadman, M.D. will certainly occupy a special place of significance. For it was during the 1950's, at a time when much of the initial impetus on the part of such luminaries as Dr. Bodog Beck and his compatriots had begun to fade that Dr. Broadman, in a medical office across the street from New York's Central Park, began to utilize the venom of the honey bee with his ailing patients. Dr. Broadman describes in the present volume that he quickly discovered that bee venom therapy was an extremely effective treatment for many arthritic and rheumatic conditions. Excited by his results which he instinctively compared to his previous forty years of using conventional approaches, he set out to convert the medical profession to the use of bee venom in selected conditions. However, as many physicians before and after him discovered, the other physicians were not interested in his work. Apparently this proved so irksome for Dr. Broadman that he redoubled his efforts to educate his colleagues. However, the more he tried to introduce them to this age-old approach which had helped so many patients down through the years, the more was he ignored and in some cases vilified.

Finally, in the early 1960's, frustrated with the refusal of the profession to listen to him, he decided to take his case directly to the patients for whom the therapy was meant. This book, the only one he ever produced on the subject, is his case for bee venom therapy. In it he presents the bulk of his resources concerning apitherapy.

The first section of the volume details many of Dr. Broadman's personal experiences in treating patients with apitherapy. In addition, he examines the history of this approach around the world. He writes about the conventional approach to the treatment of arthritic conditions which largely revolved around the use of powerful steroids. He points out, well ahead of his time, that these were potentially dangerous substances that could often do more harm than good and, at best, only suppressed the body's effort to achieve balance and homeostasis.

Unlike Dr. Beck who used honey bees in his office Dr. Broadman injected bee venom with a syringe. This was done intradermally. The author devotes a chapter to describe exactly how he practiced apitherapy. In addition, some of his articles in medical journals, which are reprinted in this volume, cover this topic.

In a sense, this book can be viewed as an update to the work pioneered in *The Bible of Bee Venom Therapy* by Dr. Beck earlier. Much of the related research performed around the world is mentioned. In addition, a bibliography of over 180 scholarly articles on bee venom therapy is provided. Much of this material may be utilized to supplement the bibliography in Dr. Beck's book.

A lengthy appendix contains many resources from diverse sources relating to apitherapy. Some of these which merit special mention include a previously untranslated presentation on bee venom by Philipp Terc, M.D., the father of apitherapy, actual correspondence from Dr. Beck whose monumental book and pivotal role in this discipline set the foundation for all who followed, and an entire section detailing Soviet research findings which are not to be found in such form elsewhere. Dr. Broadman wrote four articles about his work which were published in medical journals. These are reprinted in the appendix in their entirety.

Dr. Broadman was born in 1883. He graduated from Bellvue Medical College in 1909 in New York. He went on to practice for 57 years as a physician in New York City. By the time he died in 1966 he had assumed enough stature so that he warranted a detailed obituary in *The New York Times*. Curiously enough the writer considered his claim to fame to be his extensive library much of which was devoted to military history. In 1948 Professor William Stewart Ayers of Columbia University actually published a 35 page booklet on his collection. Dr. Broadman also was an inventor who created a process for preserving deteriorating archival materials.

According to Charles Mraz, Dr. Broadman never actually met Bodog Beck, M.D., the modern master of bee venom therapy who had died in New York in 1942. Dr. Beck had earlier written the definitive work on the subject, *The Bible of Bee Venom Therapy*, available from Health Resources Press. However, it will be evident from reading the present work that Dr. Broadman was much influenced by Dr. Beck.

Since the appearance of this work much additional evidence has surfaced to support the efficacy of bee venom therapy as propounded in this volume by Dr. Broadman. His book may be viewed as a monument to a man who put into practice his belief that it is the right of patients to be free from pain and disfiguring conditions.

Harold Goodman, D.O.
Silver Spring, Maryland

CONTENTS

FOREWORD

During my many years as a practicing physician, now concentrating on arthritic and rheumatic diseases, I have become acutely aware of the havoc these diseases have caused in pain and hardship for more than 11,000,000 people in the United States alone.

And I am even more aware that the majority of these sufferers can be cured or relieved; the means are available *now* to prevent and combat effectively these crippling diseases. These means come from the great curative value of the venom of the honey bee. Thousands have obtained relief, particularly in Europe where bee venom has been accepted for many years as the most effective cure for arthritis and rheumatism.

Resistance to bee venom as a curative has been strong in America, and it is strange that one of the most advanced countries in the world allows millions to go in agony and be crippled unnecessarily; even worse, almost all of the medical profession is completely ignorant of what bee venom can do and has done.

It is this resistance and ignorance that has forced me to write this book.

In my office, a hundred people, after relief from arthritis and rheumatism, have said to me, "Why doesn't everyone know about this treatment?"

My answer is usually one of despair and some anger. For years I have tried to publish articles in medical journals all over the country. Two have been published, but recognition for the honey bee is slow. Recently, the American Cancer Society published an article in *Cancer News* called "Does a Honey Bee Have an Answer to Cancer?" And it was gratifying to note that the Society is now doing research on the honey bee's venom, even for a disease outside of my immediate professional interests.

For most readers who are personally involved with arthritis or rheumatism, I tell you that a solution to your problems is within your grasp. It is your right to be free from pain and crippling transformations. You must demand that freedom—even if you have to "educate" your doctor to get it.

JOSEPH BROADMAN, M.D.

BEE VENOM

THE NATURAL CURATIVE
FOR ARTHRITIS AND RHEUMATISM

CHAPTER I

GOOD NEWS FOR ARTHRITICS

Arthritis and rheumatism *can* be cured. There is no need for many victims of these disabling diseases to endure painful suffering because present methods of treatment fail to bring lasting relief. A simple treatment, long used in Europe and tested in tens of thousands of cases, can bring relief and often complete cure from these dread crippling diseases. As a physician concentrating in these diseases, with publication in several reputable medical journals, I can attest to the validity of these statements even though they run counter to the current medical philosophy on the subject. But let me hasten to add, the reader needn't take my word—or my research—alone to prove my contention. There are hundreds of scientific reports, mostly from foreign countries, which demonstrate the truthfulness of what I am saying here. In fact, a thorough study of the foreign literature led me into doing my own research—with what I consider astounding results, considering the low incidence of real alleviation or cure in the rheumatoid-arthritic diseases in the U.S.

That is the good news this book brings to 11,000,000 arthritic and rheumatic sufferers in America and to those who may develop these ailments in the future. *How* and *why* this treatment has been withheld and information about it suppressed will also be revealed in these pages.

Progress is supposed to be the keynote of the twentieth century. Science, allied with technology, is constantly attaining new levels of sophistication. Our daily newspapers, our weekly and monthly publications, remind us of the strides taken in all areas of science. In the field of medicine, synthetic "wonder drugs" are discovered almost daily. Modern research does make significant progress.

Sometimes, however, research defeats its own purpose by overlooking what nature, in her inscrutable way, has provided for man. Some synthetic "curatives" fail to relieve suffering caused by disease. Often nature has already provided us with effective curatives for these diseases. *Bee venom,* the natural extract of bee poison, is just such a natural curative for arthritis and rheumatism. It surpasses all synthetic curatives in its ability to relieve these crippling diseases. *Indeed, bee venom often cures arthritis and rheumatism.*

Bee venom has long been known to help prevent arthritis and rheumatism—and to cure both when they have already developed. Dating from Greece and Rome, it has been noted that keepers of beehives are free from rheumatic pain and inflammation, either of the joints or of other parts of the body. This phenomenon has been laid to the fact that beekeepers are stung often enough to ward off these diseases. It has been established beyond much doubt, even of the established authorities, that the honeycomb contains an antiarthritic, antistiffness factor. What it is no one knows. But I am reporting facts, not their explanation, unless we can, in the best tradition of medicine, evolve a theory to explain the facts. Today bee venom is obtained *not from live bee stings, but from an isolated, purified and even standardized extract.*

Except in America, bee venom is widely accepted as a curative agent for arthritis and rheumatism. The leading medical journals of many European countries have reported on the extensive research and clinical work accomplished: different university centers in the U.S.S.R., Germany, France, Austria, Switzerland and Czechoslovakia, for example, have tested this cure. The results show that bee venom, adopted on a wide scale, can give relief or, in many cases, complete cure. Why bee venom results have not been accepted in the U.S. makes enlightening reading for those of you who still believe those persons in control of orthodox medicine are constantly searching for the cure for arthritis, no matter what the source of the cure.

The writing of this book is a matter of conscience. As a physician, I cannot rest until bee venom receives its just recognition as a curative for arthritis and rheumatism, a curative that is far more beneficial and permanent than the synthetic steroid hormones widely prescribed today—chiefly cortisone and its derivatives. When you see the mountain of evidence which the average doctor, himself, is carefully screened from seeing, then you will realize the hoax being perpetrated on the American public today. If this information shatters both your and your doctors' faith in official pronouncements, so much the better. "Official" views have tended to stifle research in many fields, not just in that of arthritis and rheumatism.

Unfortunately, many who suffer from arthritis and rheumatism have been taught to live almost helplessly resigned to their condition. An attitude of this kind reflects how completely some doctors have convinced themselves and their patients that nothing can be done. I have at my disposal and have offered to put at the disposal of other doctors two methods of treatment which many of my patients have undergone with amazing results. Many doctors have responded and have reported similar successes.

As a doctor I deplore needless human suffering and, especially, resignation to suffering. This book is not a product of my self-interest, but of my confidence in bee venom and my desire to share my knowledge with any physician interested in, or any person afflicted with, an arthritic or rheumatic condition.

There are several cogent reasons why bee venom is relatively unheard of in American medical circles. If it were not for the outmoded opinions that American medical journals retain about bee venom, particularly reports coming from *foreign* sources, and if it were not for the expensive promotion of steroids by pharmaceutical firms, then bee venom would now be helping sufferers in the U.S. to rid themselves of the centuries-old scourges known as arthritis and rheumatism. Instead, in this country, which we are constantly told is the most advanced in medical science in the whole world, most of our so-called medical leaders insist upon leading us backward and not forward. One cannot help but wonder if the real purpose of some of these medical arbiters is not more politico-economic than strictly medical. Of this, more later.

The situation is tragic and dangerous to the millions involved. For synthetic steroids have proved defective in the treatment of arthritis and rheumatism; in fact, steroid hormones such as cortisone, ACTH, Butazolidin or their derivatives have under scrutiny been challenged as practically useless by many specialists in the treatment of arthritis and rheumatism. Further, these drugs are dangerous, often causing serious side effects or death. They do not cure; neither doctors nor drug manufacturers claim they cure. These steroids were introduced originally with great fanfares of publicity with the definite implication that they would have curative value. But research has indicated they act only as analgesics; for the amount of good a patient may derive from them, aspirin is far less dangerous. In fact, as has been demonstrated in several "controlled" experiments, aspirin has proven equally as effective as the steroid hormones.

In contrast, bee venom is safer to use, causing no serious side effects or fatalities, and is simpler because it needs less medical care and one need not watch for dangerous developments. Further, it promises hope of a more lasting cure and has a more beneficial effect upon the body. Bee venom is the natural product of the honey bee. It never reacts detrimentally as do the steroid hormones now in use. (This writer believes to have proved in this book that the use of bee venom should be the preferred treatment for arthritis and rheumatism. If anyone has proof to the contrary, equaling the strength of my arguments for bee venom, it is his duty to present that proof. I would welcome such proof, if there is any.) I do not claim that bee venom will cure or improve every case of arthritis or rheumatism; badly neglected cases, those with severe irreversible joint changes, cannot be permanently benefited by any treatment now known. The only question is whether steroid hormones—the accepted major treatment—or bee venom can accomplish more under the same conditions. I think we shall demonstrate that there is no *real* choice between bee venom and the synthetic steroid hormones.

But, before we get into the actual proof, we should know more about arthritis and rheumatism and what they are. Also we should know more about the physiological effects of bee venom, what it is, and why its use has been so maligned, ignored and suppressed in the United States. The facts may shock you, but I warn you of this in advance. I tried to obtain conventional medical acceptance for bee venom therapy through normal channels. I was repulsed. Now I must carry my results to the people and to the American doctor—both of whom have been misled.

CHAPTER II

ARTHRITIS AND RHEUMATISM DEFINED

In order that the reader—both professional and lay—may not think I am offering a "crackpot" idea for the treatment of arthritis and rheumatism (such as has been propounded in the past by various persons), let me go on the record here and now with the fact that I subscribe wholeheartedly with orthodox medical science in its description of what these diseases *are* and their probable causes. This seems to me to be a matter of record, and for this reason the definitions of various forms of arthritis and rheumatism in the following few pages are taken largely from the bulletins issued by the National Institutes of Health (Division of Arthritis and Rheumatism). This subdepartment of governmental research is directly under the Department of Health, Education and Welfare.

In other words, we will go along with orthodox medicine's definition of terms and probable causes, but we fail to understand why the government scientists are so closely allied in thought with the various private groups supposedly dedicated toward finding a cure for arthritis, that they have not investigated bee venom on their own. Especially when there is so much literature on the subject.

We often call arthritis and rheumatism "diseases" but they are better described as "conditions," for they are merely local manifestations of systemic disorders and it is believed that they do not cause pathological changes in nerve tissue. The roots of these conditions are physiological rather than pathological.

Arthritis, the commonest rheumatic disease, is man's oldest known chronic affliction. The bones of the Java Ape Man and the mummies of Egypt show signs of arthritic damage. The ancient Greeks and Romans were often victims.

Rheumatic disease is called arthritis when it attacks the joints; other types, such as those that involve the muscular tissues, tendons, ligaments, bursae, etc., are grouped under the term "rheumatism." Rheumatic disease may vary from a very slight pain, stiffness or swelling to crippling and total disability. The prevalent forms of arthritis and rheumatism are discussed here.

Arthritis is the world's leading crippler. About 11,000,000 Americans suffer from arthritis and rheumatism, and 1,000,000 of these are permanently disabled. Over half the disability is in persons under 45. Rheumatic disease strikes more people than cancer, heart disease and tuberculosis combined.

Men, women and children, both young and old, can suffer rheumatic disease of one type or another. Rheumatic fever is the number one killer of children. Osteoarthritis attacks the joints of nearly everyone over 50, causing pain in one out of 20.

People with arthritis and rheumatism lose an average of

80 working days a year. Their illness costs the nation over a billion dollars annually in medical expenses, relief and lost wages.

Although the rheumatic diseases have been studied for many years the cause or causes are still unknown. Some cases follow sprains, infection or joint injury, but this is the exception rather than the rule.

Many scientists suspect viruses or bacteria, but no one has found a "rheumatic germ." Others suspect allergy. Others, disturbances of the nervous system. Still others suspect a disorder of the metabolic system—the body's means of using foods as fuel and building materials to carry on life.

We do know that emotional shock can bring on an attack of arthritis or rheumatism. And attacks often follow changes in weather. These may not be causes, but triggers that fire off an underlying condition.

The causes of arthritis and rheumatism may be manifold but, for purposes of keeping technical language to a minimum, let me say that *the main causes are due to local and relative suboxidation which comes from impaired circulation where an insufficient flow of blood and lymph produces an inadequate supply of oxygen and thus destroys living tissues.* (In short, insufficient oxygen.)

It is for this reason that the oldest cures for arthritis and rheumatism—exercise, massage, and heat—were often successful: they increased circulation and therefore oxygen to the tissues.

Sometimes arthritis and rheumatism are caused by long periods of exposure to dampness, chills, cold and drafts.

Laundry workers, for example, often contract arthritis and rheumatism.

While defective circulation and consequent insufficient oxidation are the indirect causes of arthritis and rheumatism, disturbed local metabolism and bacterial growth are the real enemies. Through faulty circulation of blood and lymph, dead cells are not eliminated and closing of the lumen (walls) of the arteries causes a calcareous, bony overgrowth which can result in osteoarthritis.

Inadequate circulation and the subsequent reduction of body resistance help bacterial growth, and bacterial growth in the joints is another contributor to the arthritic condition.

RHEUMATOID ARTHRITIS

About a third of those who visit doctors or clinics for treatment of rheumatic disease have the type known as rheumatoid arthritis. It afflicts twice as many women as men, sometimes runs in families, and usually starts between the ages of 25 and 50.

The disease causes inflammation and thickening of the lining of the joints. The lining may grow into the space and fill it. Meanwhile, the cartilage covering the ends of the bones may become eroded, and often the bones become brittle and pitted. Finally they may grow together and the joint becomes permanently fused.

Often the first signs of rheumatoid arthritis are fatigue, muscular stiffness, and loss of appetite and weight. Painful swelling then begins at one or more joints; nodules, from the size of a pea to a walnut, may appear under the skin; and muscular wasting and spasm frequently occur. The disease may affect various organs and is sometimes accompanied by fever. In some cases, despite treatment, the disease leads to chronic disability, sometimes to complete crippling.

OSTEOARTHRITIS

Degenerative joint disease, or osteoarthritis, seems to result from a combination of aging, irritation of the joints, and normal wear and tear. It is far commoner than rheumatoid arthritis, but as a rule less damaging. Older persons are the most frequent victims.

Chronic irritation of the joints is the main contributing factor. This may result from overweight, poor posture, injury, or strain from one's occupation or recreation.

The disease is characterized mainly by degeneration of joint cartilage, which becomes soft and wears unevenly. In some areas it may wear away completely, exposing the underlying bone, and thickening of the ends of the bones may occur. The remainder of the body is seldom afflicted. Except in some cases involving the hip joints, the disease causes no deformity or crippling.

Common symptoms are pain, aches, stiffness. Pain in osteoarthritis is usually experienced during use of the joints, especially finger joints and those bearing the body's weight. Enlargement of the fingers just below the last joint often occurs. Although permanent, enlargements (nodes) of this type never lead to disability.

RHEUMATIC FEVER

Of all diseases the most treacherous to children is rheumatic fever. It is the leading disease killer of youngsters between the ages of 5 and 19. Half a million children in the United States are handicapped by rheumatic fever and resulting heart damage.

Not only children but adults in great numbers are afflicted. During the Second World War, rheumatic heart disease accounted for half of the draft rejections due to diseases of the heart and circulation.

No one knows exactly what causes rheumatic fever. We do know that almost all cases begin with a streptococcus infection of the tonsils, nose or throat. Rheumatic fever strikes an average 4 per cent of the children who develop this kind of "strep" infection.

A most important recent medical advance, however, has shown that rheumatic fever is a preventable disease. Adequate medical treatment, using drugs such as sulfadiazine and penicillin, can reduce the incidence of rheumatic fever following streptococcal infections from the average 4 per cent to less than ⅕ of 1 per cent. And, although persons who have had rheumatic fever are unusually susceptible to the disease following streptococcal infection —recurrence rate has been shown to be as high as 50 per cent—the rate of recurrence can be reduced to about 2 per cent with proper use of these drugs.

Diagnosis of rheumatic fever is difficult, as there is no single reliable symptom. Danger signs, persisting for weeks or months, may be fever, pain in the limbs, nosebleeds, jerking movements of arms, legs and face. A physician can detect other signs, such as heart murmurs.

Rheumatic fever causes inflammation of many tissues of the body, including the heart, frequently damaging the heart muscle and scarring the valves. This crippling of muscles and valves produces rheumatic heart disease.

About half of the rheumatic fever patients recover completely; most of the others escape serious aftereffects.

GOUT

An arthritic disease, gout usually affects the joints of the feet, especially the big toe. A susceptibility to it is inherited, and nearly all cases occur in males. The inherited factor is a disorder of metabolism.

In the diagnosis, a chemical test is used to detect a major effect of the altered metabolism—excessive uric acid in the blood.

Gout occurs in attacks lasting days or weeks, during which the patient suffers acute joint inflammation. Between attacks he is free from symptoms. Many years after the onset, chronic arthritis may set in.

Attacks of gout usually follow minor injury, excessive eating or drinking, heavy exercise or surgical operations. However, attacks often occur with no apparent provocation.

FIBROSITIS

The commonest rheumatic condition not affecting the joints directly is fibrositis, or muscular rheumatism. It is characterized by pain, stiffness, or soreness of fibrous tissue, especially in muscles and around joints. Fibrositis within the muscles is sometimes called myositis and, when it attacks the bursae (fluid sacs in the tissue), it is known as bursitis. Lumbago is fibrositis in the lumbar region and lower part of the back.

Attacks may follow an injury, repeated muscular strain, prolonged mental tension or depression.

The condition may disappear spontaneously or respond well to treatment, but some cases persist for years. Chronic sufferers, though, are rarely crippled. Fibrositis is not a destructive, progressive disease.

Those who live in tropical or very cold countries seldom fall victim to the diseases of which we are speaking. This is probably because these people manage to keep a more or less constant body temperature, whereas "temperate" climates, with their seasonal weather changes, force alterations in body temperature which are often harmful to proper oxidation.

If you have ever wondered why arthritics and rheumatics are able to predict the coming of rain, it is because extreme humidity greatly retards the absorption and distribution of oxygen within the body, to say nothing of the elimination of carbon dioxide. Therefore, becoming listless or getting a painful disturbance in the affected area, the arthritic may often say, "It's going to rain sure as thunder; my knee is acting up again."

And if fewer young persons are arthritic, it is because in youth growth predominates along with physical activity, both of which tend to keep the organism healthy as a whole. The aged suffer greatest from arthritis and women more than men, at a ratio of approximately 5 to 1. It is believed that this is due to a lower hemoglobin content in women's blood. Arthritis is also found in so-called nervous people more than in so-called relaxed people.

All of the foregoing is informative, but from such an objective, technical discussion we can reveal nothing of the effects arthritis and rheumatism may have on the individual. Crippling transformations may be the thing we see. What goes on in the sufferer's mind, God only knows. Inability to work and consequent economic hardship may cause a man embarrassment. And what can disease do to his pride? Worst of all, perhaps, is intense physical pain—of all things the hardest to describe. It is often said that pain is man's best friend, because it is the alarm clock which wakes him up to the fact that something has gone wrong with normal bodily function. If only we could accept pain this philosophically! But we cannot. I have throughout my long career in medicine made a personal and compelling crusade against pain.

We should mention, to be honest, that the entire subject of rheumatism and arthritis is in such a confused and nebulous state that even the classification of joint diseases is still a moot point.

Physicians are groping in the dark, forced to try almost anything, alone or in combination with other medicaments, in their blind search for something with which to treat those diseased conditions. However, as we shall see, we do have a most effective agent for treatment of these painful disorders.

CHAPTER III

WHAT IS BEE VENOM AND WHEN SHOULD IT BE USED?

Now let us examine bee venom, what it is, and how it operates. We may have to be somewhat technical in places, but bear with us; it may be worth it.

Bee venom is the natural product of the honey bee, the liquid poison which the bee injects into the skin when it is angry or disturbed to create a combination of physical and chemical injury.

In case you object to the word "venom," it must be pointed out that the doctor's concept of venom or poison is a great deal different from that of the nonmedical man. We all know that poison can kill if taken in overdose; yet the quality, quantity and means of administration determine the poison's effect. Strychnine and arsenic are well-known poisons, but they are also used as curative agents. Many things we handle daily are not poisons but can be harmful. Salt, sugar and alcohol are not poisonous *per se,* but dump large quantities of them into the bloodstream and they might easily cause death.

You can even kill yourself by drinking too much water! Thus water in this quantity becomes a poison, even a lethal one. So, you see, the effect of poison is relative. There are extremely rare *instances where persons have died* from a single bee sting; others, after a hundred stings, get cured from arthritis. In medicine there is no truer saying than the old saw, what is one man's meat is another man's poison!

That bee venom actually holds the key to the salvation of approximately 11,000,000 people in the United States who suffer from arthritis and rheumatism is a fact nothing short of amazing. Even more amazing, the curative value of the venom was known in Ancient Greece. Hippocrates, the "Father of Medicine," used it and called it "Arcanum—a very mysterious remedy," and he refers to it in his eight books on medicine. So does another famous physician, Galen, 130 A.D., and also the Roman, Pliny the Elder, in his *Natural History,* written in about 14 B.C. Charlemagne, King of the Franks, 742-814, is known to have been treated with bee stings. It was thought at that time that bee stings cured all sorts of maladies and great store was laid by the venom's curative healing properties.

In the Koran, chapter XVI, 71, we find this reference to *bee venom:* "There proceeded from their bellies a liquor wherein is a medicine for men." Dr. Bodog Beck in his book *Bee Venom Therapy* (1936), used this quotation on the flyleaf.

Monfat (1600-1634) prescribed bees taken from the hive for reducing kidney "stones," the strengthening of the urinary tract and the better flow of the urine itself, as well as for a number of other conditions.

In 1859, Doctor Desjardins of France published the first scientific paper in the *Abeille Medical* (Medical Bee Journal), in which he described his bee sting treatments, which he claimed he had applied successfully in all kinds of rheumatic diseases. He even reports on two cases of skin cancer which he says he was able to cure.

In 1864, Professor Libowsky of St. Petersburg, Russia, reported in the *Courier Medical* about his success with bee stings not only in rheumatism as such, but also in cases of neuralgia as well as intermittent fever. As far back as 1850, we find reliable reports in scientific papers by many physicians about their good results treating rheumatic patients with bee stings. To mention a few: Dr. Schwabe, Germany; Dr. Hale, England; Drs. Marcy and Altschul, Germany; Dr. Goullon, France; Dr. C. Wolfe, Germany; and others.

It was not until 1879, however, that Dr. Philip Terc of Marburg, Austria, became interested in the venom of the honey bees. He was the first physician to apply bee stings in a systematic way to the treatment of rheumatic diseases. His first publication on the subject appeared in the Vienna medical press in 1888. It was the "Report About a Peculiar Connection Between the Bee Stings and Rheumatism."

Unfortunately, his own observations and all other preceding reports, found little response from his colleagues and were forgotten. Medical leaders seem to have a peculiar gift for forgetting important discoveries.

Dr. Terc, although he was laughed at throughout his career by the orthodox medical world, reported that during 25 years he had applied 39,000 bee stings to about 500 rheumatic patients without a complication, so-called side effects or fatality. Most of these patients were lastingly benefited.

Bee venom in injectable form was invented in 1928 by Dr. Franz Kretschy of Vienna. Yet, obviously, the recognition for bee venom for which Dr. Terc worked and hoped during so many years has not yet been achieved in the United States. (See Appendix H for Dr. Terc's report.)

Until comparatively recently, patients and physicians depended upon the sting of live bees for treatment. In some cases, a hundred or more stings had to be administered at one sitting.

Anyone who has been stung by *one* bee can testify to the courage of such a patient. This radical and, let's face it, wholly barbarous method was, moreover, extremely troublesome to patients.

Researchers Yoannovitch and Chahovitch wrote an interesting article which appeared in the June, 1932, number of the *Bulletin Académie de Médecine*. The subject was the treatment of experimental cancerous tumors with bee venom. They based their research on the fact that erysipelas (with consequent high fever) complicating cancer not only arrested the growth of the tumor, but greatly favored the cure of the disease and successful results, even complete cures, were reported. The favorable action of erysipelas is the result of the inflammatory phenomenon. Naturally, it would be dangerous to employ such a method, infecting patients with streptococci; the septicemia might be fatal before the tumor had a chance to recede. For this reason they never attempted such experiments.

The fact that inflammation had such pronounced effect on tumors induced them to try a substance which, when injected, would provoke inflammatory phenomena without any serious danger. Yoannovitch and Chahovitch knew that bee venom would produce such an inflammatory state, which was supposed to increase with its amount and strength. But after repeated injections, the inflammation was not so noticeable, in accordance with the laws of immunity. Cancer statistics show that people occupied in the bee industry are rarely affected by malignant growths.

Yoannovitch and Chahovitch first produced experimental cancers on the ears of a rabbit and then treated them with bee venom. Both ears developed numerous tumors, some the size of a hazelnut. The tumors were dry. Injections given daily, later on alternate days, at first with a weak solution of venom, gradually increasing the concentration. The injections were administered subcutaneously around the largest tumor. Several hours later, the inflammatory symptoms appeared and their intensity gradually increased, but the next day subsided. The tumors became soft, their bases diminished and parts fell off, followed by scar formation. The most noteworthy fact was that bee venom had an effect even on the tumors of the other ear, proving that it had not only local but *remote* and therefore, systemic, action. After the cessation of the injections, the tumors did not continue to regress, but commenced to grow again.

Their summary was: The inflammatory process produced by bee venom was not sufficient to effect the complete disappearance of the tumors, which would require a combination of the inflammatory action of the venom and injections of *some other substance,* capable of digesting the tissues of the malignant growth.

The venoms of reptiles and insects have wide usage, especially in the tropics. In Guiana it is a common practice among the natives, if one of them becomes paralyzed by drink, just to put a big ant on the victim and he will immediately regain consciousness after being stung. Stanley, in his African travels, told us that the natives pulverize dry ants, mix them with olive oil and dip their arrows into the substance, which accounts for their deadly effect. Many savage tribes poison their arrows with snake venom.

In South America, certain ants are used as an aphrodisiac, such as cantharidin ("Spanish fly"). In the seventeenth century in all European courts, Hoffman's "Vinegar of Magnanimity," made with formic acid (no relation to bee venom), was very popular. It was extensively used as a general tonic, stomachic, diuretic and aphrodisiac remedy.

Bufagin (buffaline), obtained from the secretion of the poison glands of the tropical toad *(bufo agua)*, a substance which is probably also present in the skin glands of other species of toads, proved to have heart-stimulating properties, very much like digitalis.

The study of the effects of bee stings has a decided medical interest, but in our field of investigation it has an added significance. Bee-sting injuries are, of course, very common occurrences. Medical literature abounds in a large number of published reports, which will provide us with ample material for our study. It is much more practical and also more fair to patients to acquire an accurate understanding of the effects through the study of these records than to count entirely on experiences to be gained during the course of treatments.

City physicians are only slightly interested in bee-sting injuries; on the other hand, in the country this type of injury might have considerable importance. To my knowledge, there is so far no complete textbook available on the subject.

The sting of the bee is nothing else but a poisoned

wound, a combination of a physical and a chemical injury. Accordingly, we must consider and distinguish between, first, the more or less painful mechanical injury caused by a barbed sting gradually penetrating the skin; and second, a burning, extremely excruciating sensation which accompanies the injury and is produced by the chemical action of a caustic venom which progressively irritates new nerve filaments of the skin. It is a characteristic, interrupted, lancinating pain.

The local physiological effect of the bee sting is generally violent inflammation, hyperemia (edema) caused by the escape of blood plasma and a circulatory hardening, in the center of which is often a local destruction of tissue.

At first a pale "papule" forms. We call it the "wheal," and this gradually extends in circumference with more or less rapidity, depending, of course, on the strength and quantity of the venom and on the individual sensitivity of the victim. In the center, a little red spot and sometimes a minute drop of blood are visible as the direct result of the mechanical injury. Around the wheal the hyperemic (excessive blood) tissues become harder and increase both in size and elevation. The area is painful on pressure but not very sensitive to superficial touch. There is always a certain numbness in the center on account of the anesthetizing effect of the local infiltration.

The general systemic effects of bee venom on the organism are extremely variable and complex. They demand careful consideration. There is no possible way to judge, still less to put a standard from which we could foretell, the consequences from the stings, or vice versa. A very few cases end fatally as the result of only one sting while others, where hundreds of stings were inflicted, might not show any ill effects. The modifying circumstances are so manifold that it is almost impossible even to attempt an explanation of certain phenomena. We continually meet new, unexpected and strange incidents. The effects of the majority of bee-sting injuries are unquestionably normal, but then again we are often confronted with plenty of surprises—even miracles.

A person sensitive to bee stings is likely to exhibit the following symptoms within several minutes: chills, high temperature, diffuse perspiration, headache, vertigo, dizziness, nausea, vomiting, diarrhea, great thirst, laryngeal and chest constriction, extreme weakness and even unconsciousness. The pulse is rapid. Later a general itching, hives, and in places edematous swelling may develop all over the body.

We repeat: These alarming symptoms occur only in those very few persons allergic to bee stings. *In actual practice we have a simple test to determine whether or not a person is sensitive to bee venom.*

Bee venom is a water-clear liquid with a sharp, bitter taste and aromatic odor (comparable to ripe bananas), having a distinctly acid reaction.

It is easily soluble in water and acids, almost insoluble in alcohol. It contains 30 per cent solid matter. The venom dries easily in ordinary room temperature. Drying will convert it into a gum-like substance, without any loss of potency. It withstands 100° C. temperature for ten days without losing any of its power. Cold, even freezing, does not destroy its effect.

Bee venom, however, is easily destroyed by oxidizing substances: potassium permanganate, potassium sulphate; halogen elements—chlorine and bromine—destroy it very quickly; the effect of iodine is much slower. Alcohol possesses a strong and quick destructive effect on the venom.

Bee venom has no effect on uninjured skin, but it has powerful effects upon mucous membranes, except upon those of the alimentary tracts. The gastric and intestinal ferments will quickly destroy it. Because of this fact, bee venom, if taken internally, is usually ineffective. On the eye and nose membrane surfaces it produces an especially strong effect.

If preserved from moisture, bee venom will keep for years. In glycerin, it keeps indefinitely without losing toxicity.

F. Flury, world-famous toxicologist of the University of Wuerzburg, following in the footsteps of Langer, in 1920 found the venom to contain the following substances: tryptophan, choline, glycerin, phosphoric acid, palmitic acid, fatty acid (noncrystallizable), a volatile acid (likely butyric acid) and a non-nitrogenous substance. Flury was convinced that the last-named substance is the pharmacologically active and the physiological effective component of the venom.

Flury felt justified in concluding that bee venom was a complex substance, a combination between an albumin-free sapotoxin of animal origin and a poison, such as one of the cantharidin group. The active agent was always in combination with *lecithin.* The active agent is *not formic acid* as had been previously and erroneously reported. In fact, bee venom contains no formic acid. Yet this is the substance which was used in most of the so-called experiments in the United States which have pronounced "bee venom" worthless. See reports of Dr. Walter Alvarez in Chapter 7 in which he specifically states that formic acid was used—as though it were *still* considered the active ingredient in bee venom. Sometimes a medical man is slower in learning the truth than one might reasonably expect. But, of course, that may not be anything other than his authoritarian training which starts in medical school and usually lasts throughout his life. Few people realize how hard it is to escape one's teachings and initial orientation in any field—not just medicine.

Therefore it is with some reluctance that I must present to you the most cogent and, I believe, scientifically valid explanation of bee venom and how it works. I say with some reluctance because—although as a scientist I accept scientific information from any source—nevertheless it is unfashionable and one is rendered suspect if one acknowledges that the Soviets are far ahead in both theory and practice in *any* phase of scientific endeavor.

Yet as a scientist, I would be unfaithful to the credo of science if I attempted to cover up the Soviet scientists' paramount achievements in the field of bee venom. I do believe you cannot suppress facts for any great length of time no matter where they originate.

Herewith follows a paper delivered in Rome, Italy, in September, 1958, by Professor N. M. Artemov of Gorki University, U.S.S.R. I have left it in its exact language. The medical terms are not difficult. Read it and you will get a clear picture (as far as possible at the moment) as to *why* bee venom is effective.

THE BIOLOGICAL PRINCIPLES OF THE APPLICATION OF BEE VENOM IN MEDICINE

"The therapeutic application of both bee venom and its preparations is effected so far empirically, without a sufficient theoretical base. That is why the development of a medicobiological theory of the bee venom effect on the healthy and the diseased organism is a problem of particular importance. This theory must throw light upon all known facts from the special point of view and make clear the complicated symptom-complex of poisoning as well as the therapeutic properties of bee venom.

"The author of the present article succeeded in putting forward an hypothesis meeting the above-mentioned requirements on the basis of the experimental data he obtained in his laboratory. He further examined his hypothesis from the biological and evolutionary point of view. The bee sting and bee venom are known to be fit to protect the bee against its chief enemies—the mammals—who closely interacted with bees in the process of evolution. As a result, the venom developed as a factor acting upon the most vulnerable and important systems of the organism (nervous system, blood) on the one hand, while on the other, mammals have developed the ability to react to venom by mobilizing all their protective forces and by increasing their resistance to it. As a result the venom has become the natural adequate stimulus of protective reactions of the [mammalism] organism.

"In fact the analysis of the symptom complex of poisoning with bee venom gives us the opportunity of subdividing its symptoms into two categories: (a) symptoms depending upon the disintegration of cells and organs or the inactivation of some biochemical systems, (b) symptoms associated with the realization of the protective reactions. Such symptoms as haemolysis [red blood cell destruction] and cytolysis [cellular destruction], muscular contractions, the blockade or nervous synapse and inactivation of enzymes (e.g., dehydrase) belong to the first category. The system of the mutually associated symptoms which indicate 'general adaptation syndrome' belongs to the second category.

"Among these symptoms are the shock developing at the beginning of the poisoning, the characteristic variations in blood, the increasing permeability of the blood vessels, the excitation of the pituitary-adrenocortical system and the change of reactivity in the organism; in particular, the increase of resistance to the venom. All of them have been carefully examined and studied in detail. It has been evidenced that the protective inhibition occurring in the cerebral cortex of animals after the injection of non-lethal doses of the venom, should be also included in the second category."

According to the above-mentioned hypothesis, the therapeutic properties of the venom are quite obvious. They are associated with the mobilization of the organism's protective forces—in particular with the increase of the internal secretion of the pituitary and the adrenal cortex with the subsequent reconstruction of the organism's reactivity. For this reason bee venom is especially effective in cases of rheumatic disease and allergies which are characterized by abnormal reactivity and which cannot be cured by using cortisone and ACTH.

This hypothesis has made it possible to give a rational

interpretation and classification of the poisoning symptoms which so far were merely enumerated without disclosing their correlation and development. We can now predict still unknown symptoms and work out a rational treatment in the case of venom poisoning.

Finally, with the help of this hypothesis, it is possible to explain the "immunity" of beekeepers, the nature of which still remains obscure. Now it has been proved that the immunity cannot be regarded as a result of specific antitoxins since the "mellitin," the active base of the venom, does not possess antigenic properties. In my opinion, beekeepers' immunity is nothing but a resistance stage in the "general adaptation syndrome."

Thus we see bee venom's curative powers can best be explained by its stimulating effect on blood and blood vessels—in short, its ability to increase circulation. After a bee venom injection, blood cells transmigrate into the tissues. The venom opens the capillary walls, thus allowing the body a better elimination of waste matter as well as increased metabolism which enriches the supply of oxygen within the body. Better circulation and intensified oxidation also help to destroy bacterial growth, in this way enabling a normal physical state to replace the pathological condition.

Bee venom attacks the contributing causative factors of arthritis and rheumatism; it does not merely treat symptoms as do the so-called "wonder" drugs. It attacks at the cellular level where every disease begins. This is important because relieving pain or treating the outward manifestations of any disease does not indicate in any way that the disease has been removed. Folklore has it that the ostrich sticks his head in the sand when it is afraid or cornered by an enemy. True, the ostrich cannot see the enemy, but that does not eliminate him nor make the ostrich any safer. And just as the ostrich may get dirt in his eyes by "treating only the symptoms," so are there added dangers in using steroids. Bee venom contains none of these dangers which can cause death.

Another curative factor of the venom is known as its *neurotoxic* effect. This means that the venom, creating a slight paralytic or sedative effect on nerve centers—not, however, on blood vessels—acts as a tonic both physically and mentally.

And so our friend, the bee, does man a greater service than he is ever likely to realize as he goes on his rounds collecting pollen and nectar from flowers and turning the nectar into honey in his mysterious, instinctive way.

Until recently, patients and physicians depended upon the stings of live bees for treatment. As we have stated, in some cases, a hundred or more stings had to be administered at one sitting. Often, too, the bee venom supply would run out, especially during the winter months when the need was greatest.

Today, as we have said previously, the venom is isolated, purified and even standardized. Available in injectable form, it may be safely administered without noticeable pain. Only in cases among women with a history of glandular malfunction does the treatment work more slowly. Experience has also demonstrated that patients with syphilis, tuberculosis or gonorrhea are highly allergic to bee venom. In such cases it should never be used. It is important, not only to treat cases correctly, but also to select them carefully.

Thanks to the method devised by the late Dr. G.

Laughton-Scott of London, England (See Appendix B), and bee venom, the physician now has at his disposal two distinct methods of treatment which are applicable to the many types of rheumatic diseases, whether rheumatoid or otherwise. The doctor can conveniently administer both these methods with very little discomfort for the patient. Moreover, *any* general practitioner, no matter where he is located, can apply these methods, for the technique of treatment is mastered easily in a few hours.

As soon as suspicion arises that we may be facing a case of rheumatic nature of known or unknown origin, treatment with bee venom should be started. In this simple precaution alone—early treatment—lies the patient's best chance for early and complete recovery. In many of the newer cases, where no joint changes have yet occurred, improvement and recovery are often so rapid that it is difficult for the average person, even a physician, to believe it. Although some rheumatic conditions are not easily differentiated in the early stages, the physician should not delay the treatment. An error made in early diagnosis would not hurt the patient but would afford him a degree of safety for complete, early recovery. In the nonarthritic types of rheumatism, however, we do not deal with possible joint changes. We use Scott's method in certain cases of severe joint changes when bee venom does not bring relief.

Both methods employ injections. The differences lie in the application (systemic or local) and in the substance injected (bee venom or salicylate compounds). Whereas the Scott method uses local injections with local effects only, the bee venom is injected intradermally and acts systemically. Another difference between the two methods amounts to this: while the Scott method must treat each rheumatic lesion separately, the bee venom, through its systemic action, may affect several lesions simultaneously.

The Scott method has been elaborately verified and authenticated in England. For 20 years, Dr. Scott did research on nonrheumatoid arthritis and rheumatism. The result was a new therapy for these diseases, but not for rheumatoid arthritis. (Briefly, the Scott method utilizes compounds of salicylate acids [aspirin] and camphor. These are injected directly into the afflicted joints.)

After Dr. Scott presented his findings to the London Medical Society, the Society appointed a Special Committee of well-known rheumatologists, headed by Dr. C. B. Heald of London, to investigate Dr. Scott's reports and therapy. For two years this committee made an extensive study of Dr. Scott's findings. The work was split into four parts, each part establishing a treatment center in a different section of England. Each center, with a member of the committee presiding, treated about 50 patients. Since the Scott method is intended solely for nonrheumatoid rheumatic conditions, the committee decided to use it exclusively on fibrosities and to bar all other medication during the course of treatment given each patient.

Before writing their joint report for the parent body, the committee assessed each case on a uniform basis; after six months each case was specifically reassessed by each of the four committee members *independently*. The clinical value of such a method of testing and evaluation requires no emphasis. Of nearly 200 patients treated, the committee reported that 78.5 per cent benefited from treatment. The committee also stressed the independence of the investigation, in which Dr. Scott played no part beyond personally administering the treatments to each patient to ensure the use of the proper technique. The findings of the committee, which were highly favorable to Scott's method, were published in the *Lancet,* the official journal of the British Medical Association.

After I read the *Lancet* report, I went to London to work and study with Dr. Scott. I have since applied his method to my own practice in New York. But would you not think in the face of all this scientific evidence that American medicine would eagerly seize on the Scott method? No, indeed, the various orthodox agencies here ignored this great work. However, they are still collecting millions in an "all out" attempt—they say—to find causes and cures for arthritis and rheumatism.

To my knowledge, I am the only physician in the U.S. who uses the Scott method where it is applicable. I have had many successes with it, but we cannot enumerate them here. We must stick to the simple bee venom treatment.

The first treatment with bee venom includes a test for allergy to the medication, a test so simple that any physician performs it in seconds. If there are no allergic reactions within 15 minutes, the patient can undergo any amount of required treatment without danger of complications. The technique itself is simple. Any physician can readily grasp it either through reading this book or through observation at my clinic.

The principle of the bee venom treatment is saturation of the patient with the medication. Saturation is reached when all wheals fuse to form one mass, called a *plaque.* Saturation with bee venom means immunity which, although not permanent, can be repeated every three to five years. As far as the dosage is concerned, it should be adequate and gradually increased, either daily or every other day, depending on the individual case. Two or three months after the first treatments are concluded, several extra treatments may be given which will assure a lasting result.

However, each case has to be carefully considered. This is so because contraindications can occur.

Severe kidney involvements, *albuminuria* (too much albumin in the blood) demand vigilance and discretion. Cases with cardiovascular complications, as a rule, are delicate and if such pathological conditions are advanced, bee venom treatments are absolutely contraindicated. To this group belong: *myocarditis, angina pectoris, arteriosclerosis, aneurism of the aorta* and, in short, any chronic cardiovascular condition. However, rheumatic inflammation of the heart, *endocarditis* and *pericarditis*—acute or chronic—are not only *not* contraindicated but are suitable cases for treatment.

Of course, I repeat, watch out for the trio, the *"bête noire"* of bee venom therapy: tuberculosis, syphilis and gonorrhea. Fortunately, these diseases are not as prevalent as they once were, thanks to modern treatments. Even rarer are those in the later stages. Severe diabetes is generally a contraindication, but diabetics only rarely require intense treatments, as arthritis among them is exceptional.

All arthritis caused by glandular imbalance, such as *climacteric* arthritis, does not respond readily to bee venom treatment, as the progress of the producing causes remains unbroken. A history of rheumatism, of course, is a peremptory requirement.

The ailments listed below are amenable to bee venom therapy (see Glossary for definitions): muscular rheumatism, myalgia, myositis, fibrositis, neuritis, neuralgia, migraine, trigeminal neuralgia, sciatica, acute rheumatic fever and endocarditis, acute and chronic osteoarthritis, acute and chronic rheumatoid arthritis, arthritis deformans, spondylitis (Bechterew), gout, chronic surgical inflammation of the soft and bony tissues, rheumatic iritis and motor paralysis.

MUSCULAR RHEUMATISM, MYALGIA, MYOSITIS

The ailments in this category yield quickly to bee venom therapy, as the pathological conditions produced by ischemia and anoxemia are easily corrected by the powerful hemorrhagic effect of the venom.

The marvelous cures of paralytic cases reported by the various continental beehive "clinics" could be explained as motor paralysis afflictions due to some interference with the blood supply of certain parts of the nervous system (Volkmann's paralysis). Good results from bee venom in such instances are obtained rapidly. They are often amazing.

NEURITIS, NEURALGIA, MIGRAINE

The rapidity with which results are secured in this group almost equals that achieved in muscular rheumatism which disorders, as stated in the preceding subdivision, yield readily to bee venom treatments.

ACUTE RHEUMATIC FEVER AND ENDOCARDITIS

The maladies of this group present a fruitful field for bee venom treatments. Terc and Keiter often mention the fact that bee venom can be rightfully considered a specific in rheumatic fever and endocarditis.

The treatments are administered on alternate days, starting with low concentration, increasing the number of wheals by two or three, or even more, stepping up to high concentration. On the days when no injections are given, Kretschy suggested administering antipyretics (fever-reducing drugs) if the temperature is high but, when it approaches normal, only the venom should be used.

ACUTE AND CHRONIC ARTHRITIS

The typical case of rheumatoid arthritis is much more resistant to treatment than muscular rheumatism, neuritis, or even rheumatic fever or endocarditis rheumatica. The response is much slower. Complete immunization of the patients is essential; they must be "saturated" with bee venom. Traumatic arthritis, on the other hand, responds very rapidly. *Bechterew's disease, spondylitis deformans* is included in this group. The results with bee venom are very good. The distressing characteristic symptoms of this disease, such as profuse perspiration, will quickly disappear. The pressure exerted by the compression and irritation of the nerve roots soon shows a distinct improvement and also there is freer mobility of the spine. Patients all state that they feel "looser."

Acute and chronic gout also belong under this heading. Reports about the results obtained in this class are very favorable, depending, of course, on the chronicity and character of the case.

ARTHRITIS DEFORMANS

The reactions produced in treating arthritis *deformans* differ absolutely from those obtained in all other rheumatic ailments. In arthritis *deformans,* the first reactions appear much sooner, not only the local but also the general and focal. We find swellings in the joints during the reactions, but without any improvement. The postreactive and succeeding nonreactive stages are also extremely short. The reactive and nonreactive phases alternate frequently during protracted treatments.

While in other groups we can fairly predict the approximate duration of a nonreactive state, in arthritis *deformans* this is impossible. Therefore, it is advisable to proceed slowly because we cannot foretell when the reactions will suddenly appear. The treatments are usually long because we must proceed leisurely, and the improvement will be correspondingly delayed. A rapid advance may aggravate conditions.

Women are often subject to arthritis *deformans.* If it is caused by changes or other glandular disturbances, the treatments will be less favorable. (It is a peculiar fact that many arthritis *deformans* sufferers are hypersensitive to tuberculin—the substance used to determine if the patient has tuberculosis.)

RHEUMATIC IRITIS

Rheumatic iritis represents rather painful and distressing complications of rheumatism and arthritis and, according to several authors, responds to bee venom therapy, even when all other remedies have failed.

But it is in Soviet Russia—apart from my own necessarily limited experiments in this country—where the final good word about the efficacy of bee venom is being written. We must face the fact that the U.S.S.R., in *medicine* at least, is not hampered by tradition or by the need to make money from medical findings. If, for instance, a substance such as cortisone does not work in treating arthritis or rheumatism, the treatment is discarded. It does not take the agony and the failures of millions of arthritics to prove to *their* orthodoxy that better means of treatment should be found instead of promoting the old failures—no matter how much the failures may be stockpiled in the pharmaceutical laboratories and crying for distribution.

As a recent example of the way American scientists are treated when they develop something which runs counter to the current orthodox fad, let me cite the case of Dr. Albert Sabin. By the time you read this, Dr. Sabin's oral vaccine for polio will be available in the U.S., and you will probably see a big propaganda buildup in the medical, and therefore the public, press extolling the values of the oral vaccine. It *could* have been extolled several years before.

In spite of many deaths attributed to the Salk vaccine (improperly manufactured), the Sabin vaccine (with no deaths attributed to it) was shunted aside in favor of Salk's. In time the failure of the Salk vaccine to overcome paralytic polio became apparent: first two, then three, and finally four shots were considered necessary to protect one against polio—all necessitating expenses of the doctor's time and the cost of the injections themselves. Meanwhile, the pharmaceutical houses which manufactured the Salk vaccine were making multi-millions from the sale of the vaccine. Even though the vaccine had been developed by Dr. Salk who had been the recipient of public donations from citizens who had contributed to the "March of Dimes"—the National Polio Foundation's method of raising funds. Salk's discovery was announced with a great fanfare of publicity, in direct contradistinction to medical ethics—so the medical authorities tell us when such a discovery is released seemingly without their being "in" on the releasing.

Meanwhile, back at the unaccepted medical ranch, Dr. Sabin (and several other medical scientists who had also developed an oral vaccine which necessitated the taking of only one to three pills for practically complete protection) was seething.

As everyone now knows, Dr. Sabin took his polio vaccine to Soviet Russia where it was well received. It was given to about 80,000,000 Russians—also many other foreign countries tested it on millions of people. It proved so efficacious that finally the United States Public Health Department had to recognize it and offer it to the American public. The U.S. Public Health Department announced it was the "safety factor" which held up their recognition of the Sabin vaccine—though the record shows that Sabin's vaccine has killed no one.

In other words, the U.S. government's medical agencies are so closely tied in with the pharmaceutical industries and the orthodox medical groups that they would still promote the sale of the Salk vaccine even when they admitted the oral vaccine was better.

Thus it was not until the fall of 1961—when the polio season was conveniently over—that Dr. Sabin's oral vaccine was accepted by the A.M.A. and the U.S.P.H.S.

CHAPTER IV

FACTS FROM MY RECORDS: THE CASE HISTORIES

Now it is time for us to get down to actual case histories —that is, people who have been cured or helped by my injections of bee venom. (The thousands of cases in foreign countries who have been benefited, we will report in other chapters and in the Appendix.)

These are persons who have come to me in spite of the adverse propaganda against bee venom. These are people who somehow do not fall for the slick medical propaganda which tells them that bee venom is useless in the treatment of arthritis. These are the people whose records you will see below. I have purposely left these records in their original medical terminology so that no professional reader can say the records were altered in the slightest degree in order to "popularize"—and therefore possibly exaggerate— the case for bee venom therapy. I believe most layman readers, particularly those who suffer from arthritis and have read anything about it, will understand the language. (A Glossary of medical terms used in this book is published in the Appendix.)

Unless otherwise indicated, the improvement in these

patients has lasted up until the present writing (September, 1961).

CASE 1: P.F., an 84-year-old male, was examined in April, 1952, with a history of a severe, burning pain in his left arm for the past six months. He showed fibrositic nodules in the biceps of the arm corresponding with the localized tenderness. Past treatments with cortisone, massage and diathermy were of no avail. The diagnosis was rheumatic fibrositis of the left biceps. The patient received four injections, without reaction, and was discharged free of symptoms.

CASE 2: M.F., a 40-year-old male, gave a history of pain in his back which increased with bad weather and on sitting. There was an area of tenderness in the region of the fourth and fifth lumbar vertebrae. The diagnosis was osteoarthritis of those vertebrae, and this was confirmed by X-ray. After eight injections he was discharged and has remained free of symptoms.

CASE 3: M.S., a 35-year-old female, was seen in October, 1952, with a history of very severe pains in the cervical region for the past six months. All previous treatment failed to give relief. She presented areas of deep-seated tenderness on both sides of the neck at the level of the third cervical vertebra, which was diagnosed as brachial neuritis. The patient was given six injections on each side, after which she was discharged free of symptoms, and has remained so to date. (This woman is divorced with a little boy to care for. She works during the day while preparing in night school for the stage. She became so despondent over her condition that she contemplated suicide. When she was told that injections were indicated, she cried bitterly "because," she said, "every injection I took only made me worse.") It required much effort on the part of the gentleman who brought her—who was himself cured by me—to induce her to take the treatments.)

CASE 4: D.A., a 40-year-old male, was examined in November, 1952, with a history of pain in his back and gluteal region for one year, with frequent recurrence. He presented areas of acute tenderness in the gluteal region and over the fourth and fifth lumbar and first sacral vertebrae. The Lasègue test was positive; ankle jerks were absent. Some sensory loss was found on the outer surface of the legs and soles. Diagnosed as rheumatic sciatica, the patient received two injections and was discharged. He has remained free of symptoms since.

CASE 5: F.V., a 60-year-old female, was seen in November, 1952, with a long history of severe pains in both knees as well as severe pains in her back. She was unable to walk and was bedridden. The knees were tender with considerable swelling in both. There was limited motion, especially on flexion. She had areas of tenderness over the fourth and fifth lumbar vertebrae. Osteoarthritis of both knees and of the fourth and fifth lumbar vertebrae was confirmed by X-ray. All four lesions were treated simultaneously, with six injections to each, after which she was discharged. She has remained free of symptoms to date and is able now to walk any desired distance. (Ironically, when this patient told her previous physician that she felt entirely relieved and that she was discharged from treatment, he replied "then it could not have been arthritis.")

CASE 6: J.R., a 43-year-old male, was treated in January, 1953, for distressing pain in his left knee for the past six years. For the past two years the pain never left him entirely. There were areas of tenderness in the gastrocnemius muscle, well localized, which were diagnosed as rheumatic fibrositis of that muscle, and the patient was given six injections. He was discharged and he has remained free of symptoms since.

CASE 7: R.R., a 32-year-old male, was examined because of pain in his left elbow for six months. He showed an area of tenderness in the extensor carpi radialis longus of that side, consistently localized, which was diagnosed as a rheumatic fibrositis. The patient was given seven treatments, after which he was discharged and he has remained free of symptoms to date.

CASE 8: S.B., a 45-year-old male, presented himself in May, 1953, with a history of pain in his left knee for the past six months. Eleven injections of cortisone brought no relief. He had pain and difficulty on walking. Flexion of that knee was limited. He had a warm joint, slightly swollen, with pain upon flexion. Diagnosed as osteoarthritis of the left knee, he received six injections and was discharged, remaining free of symptoms since.

CASE 9: A.H., a 28-year-old female, was seen in May, 1953, stating that for several weeks she has had pain in her left knee, especially when walking and in bad weather. She had a swollen knee, warm and tender on palpation, with slightly limited flexion. The diagnosis of osteoarthritis of the left knee was confirmed by X-ray and the patient was given one injection only. She insisted that she felt completely relieved and would take no more, but promised to return for monthly examinations. She has remained free of symptoms.

CASE 10: I.D., a 38-year-old female, was treated in May, 1953, for pain in her right arm extending to her shoulder and neck. She could not raise that arm and had difficulty at work. After a diagnosis of rheumatic fibrositis of the right deltoid was established, she received six treatments and was discharged free of symptoms with normal function restored.

CASE 11: A.R., a 33-year-old male, was examined in August, 1953, with a five-year history of pain in the back. He had difficulty in straightening up after sitting down in a chair. Bending was painful. The pain interfered with his work and with his sleep. Palpation did not disclose any definite signs of tenderness in any location. Roentgenologic examination showed definite osteoarthritis of second, third, fourth and fifth lumbar vertebrae. Patient was given six treatments to each lesion and discharged free of symptoms. He has remained so to date.

CASE 12: J.B., a 70-year-old female, was examined in February, 1953; she stated that for about five years she has had recurrent pain in her back which gave her considerable trouble. She has had difficulty in walking and inability to sleep. At time of examination her pain was much worse. There was an area of tenderness in the region of the fourth and fifth lumbar vertebrae. The pain extended to the right buttock and down the leg. The Lasègue test was positive. Dorsiflexion of foot increased the pain. The diagnosis was made of rheumatic sciatica. Only two injections were given and the patient was discharged. She had been free of symptoms until she died of an unrelated illness.

CASE 13: F.R., a 61-year-old female, was examined in August, 1953, with a history of pain in the gluteal region, radiating down the leg and thigh. She could not work at all, because she could not stand even for short periods. Walking was painful, as was rising. Examination disclosed tenderness along the course of the sciatic nerve, and along the lower lumbar vertebrae. The Lasègue test was positive. Dorsiflexion of the foot increased the pain. Ankle jerks were absent. Diagnosis was made of rheumatic sciatica and osteoarthritis of the fourth and fifth lumbar vertebrae, the last confirmed by roentgenogram. Three treatments were given for sciatica and six treatments for the osteoarthritis, and the patient was discharged. She has remained free of symptoms to date.

CASE 14: R.M., a 42-year-old male, was examined in August, 1953, with a five-year history of pain in his back. He could not sleep and bad weather affected him very much. He had difficulty when walking and rising from a chair. Tenderness was found in the lower back and in the glutei muscles, radiating down the leg. The Lasègue test was positive. Dorsiflexion of the foot test was positive. Diagnosis was made of rheumatic sciatica and osteoarthritis of the lower lumbar vertebrae. Roentgenologic examination confirmed the presence of osteoarthritis of the third, fourth and fifth lumbar vertebrae. One injection was given for the sciatica and six injections for the arthritis, and the patient was discharged free of symptoms. He has remained free of symptoms since.

CASE 15: J.C., a 55-year-old female, was examined in October, 1953, with a history of severe pain in the back for some years, which suddenly had become much worse, extending down the thigh. She has had difficulty with her work, and has experienced difficulty in walking. The cold weather made her condition worse. Examination showed definite tenderness in the glutei muscles, and some tenderness in the thigh. The Lasègue test was positive. Diagnosis was made of rheumatic sciatica and two injections were given; the patient was discharged free of symptoms, and has remained so.

CASE 16: M.F., a 55-year-old male, was examined in November, 1954, with a history of pain in the back for about two years. He had to give up work on several occasions because of pain and difficulty in walking, and when rising from a chair. Sitting was painful and bad weather increased his symptoms. Examination showed an area of tenderness in his back along the fourth and fifth lumbar vertebrae, and also a tenderness over the right sacroiliac joint. The Mennell test increased the pain on the affected side, and the Hopkins test did the same. The Lasègue test was negative. Diagnosis was made of osteoarthritis of lumbar vertebrae and of the right sacroiliac joint disease, which was confirmed by roentgenogram. Six treatments were given to the fourth and fifth lumbar vertebrae, and four treatments for the sacroiliac joint; the patient discharged as free of symptoms and has remained so to date.

CASE 17: B.H., a 41-year-old female, was examined in December, 1954, with a history of severe pain in the back since early youth. For the past four years the pain has been more severe. Bending was very difficult, if not impossible. Walking was painful and bad weather increased her pain. She could not sleep, nor straighten up after sitting down. The examination showed areas of tenderness along the lumbar spine. Diagnosis was made of osteoarthritis of lumbar vertebrae, and the roentgenogram confirmed the diagnosis for the third, fourth and fifth lumbar. The patient was given three treatments to each lesion and discharged free of symptoms. She has remained so.

CASE 18: CH.Z., a 65-year-old male, came to see me March 31, 1954, with a history of severe pain in his left shoulder for the past three years. Repeated treatments were of no avail. Examination disclosed tender areas and trigger spots over the left shoulder. X-ray did not show any other condition present and a diagnosis of fibrositis was made. Patient received six treatments, when he felt perfectly well and he was discharged. He has remained well since and has so reported from time to time.

CASE 19: G.D., a 55-year-old male, came to see me January 4, 1955, with an acute pain in his right leg. The pain radiated up and down so that he could not walk, sit or stand. Examination disclosed a very tender area about the right knee and a diagnosis of periarticular fibrositis of the right knee was made. After the first injection patient was completely relieved and able to return to work. He received two more injections and was discharged. He has been free of symptoms to date.

CASE 20: B.S., a 57-year-old female, consulted me on March 1, 1955, with a history of pain in her right shoulder. At night the pain was much worse. The shoulder was very sensitive to cold wind or breezes. Examination showed definite trigger points around the joints and the diagnosis of fibrositis was made. Patient received two treatments and discontinued further treatments. She reported three years later that she had been completely well ever since.

CASE 21: J.A., a 51-year-old male, was seen on November 17, 1956. He stated that for the past month he had been very ill and in severe pain, first from his right and left foot, later from his left knee, followed by involvement of his right knee. At that time all his symptoms were worse. He was brought to the office in a wheelchair. All previous treatments with cortisone were without results. Examination showed a very ill person with a very swollen and painful right knee. The left knee and both feet were less acute, but swollen and painful. Temperature 102.5°. ESR was 85 mm. X-ray showed a clouding of both knees due to synovitis, and a clouding of all joints in the feet and ankles due to synovitis. There was a moderate decalcification of the bones of the left foot. Diagnosis was made of an acute rheumatoid arthritis and bee venom therapy was begun. Patient responded well from the start. Two weeks later he was already able to get around on crutches. At the end of his second course, on February 6, 1957, he was discharged as completely recovered. He has remained well to date.

CASE 22: A.G., a 47-year-old male, was seen in June, 1955, with a history of acute illness since early in February, when he suffered severe pain in his right foot, which quickly spread to his right knee and right hip. Could not walk, was bent, had difficulty in sitting down or rising except under severe pain. The cortisone he had received did not help at all. Examination revealed an acutely ill patient with a tender and swollen right foot, right knee and right hip. Could not stand erect, walk or sit down. Temperature 102°. ESR 100 mm. X-ray showed narrowing and almost complete obliteration of the right sacroiliac joint, associated with irregular sclerosis of the articular margins. Diagnosis of acute rheumatoid arthritis was made and bee venom was started. Patient did well and was discharged as well on December 20, 1955. He has been well to date.

CASE 23: B.J., a 39-year-old female, seen on December 30, 1954, with a history that for one year she had had pain in her right knee. It kept her awake and she could not bend it. It was swollen and it troubled her when walking, especially down stairs. The pain was sharper when sitting down or getting up. Examination showed a swollen knee with limited motion, tender and with severe pain on flexion. She was in constant pain. X-ray showed a clouding of the knee joint and a thickening of the synovium, particularly in the suprapatelar region. Diagnosis was made of rheumatoid arthritis and bee venom was given. The patient responded very promptly and on April 21, 1955, she was discharged. Patient has been well to date.

CASE 24: I.N., a 50-year-old female, was seen in March, 1955. Her statement was that five years earlier she had her first attack of pain in the right hand, followed by pain in the left arm and right foot. Gradually, it spread to the left foot and other joints. Now in both feet. At time of examination, she had difficulty in sitting, rising and walking. Most joints were involved, with difficulty in mobility, stiffness, flexion and rotation. ESR was 60 mm. X-ray showed punched out areas in fingers and toes. Diagnosis was made of chronic gout and bee venom therapy commenced. With some vacations from treatment between courses, the therapy was concluded on January 20, 1956 at patient's request.

CASE 25: A.F., a 60-year-old male, was seen on July 8, 1956. He stated that for four months he had been suffering from pain in his back. This extended to his thighs and knees, followed by pain in both shoulders and hands and finally the neck became painful. Had difficulty in sleeping, walking and could not turn his head. At time of examination, patient had difficulty in bending and walking and turning. He showed deep-seated painful trigger points on both sides of neck. The pain in the back extended from the lumbar region to the legs of both sides. Lasègue test was positive; dorsiflexion increased the pain; ankle jerks were absent; some sensory loss was found on the outer surface of the legs and soles. Diagnosis was made of bilateral brachial neuralgia and bilateral sciatica. Bee venom was administered and response was prompt. After 13 injections patient was discharged on July 21, 1956. He has remained well to date.

CASE 26: D.C., a 45-year-old female, was seen on July 12, 1956, with a history of pain in her neck for ten years and difficulty in rotating head. Pain was worse at times, preventing sleep. Lately she had had pains in her right thigh and foot. All symptoms were getting worse. Examination disclosed deep-seated tenderness on right side of neck, tenderness in right gluteal region, radiating down to the thigh and leg. Lasègue test was positive. Dorsiflexion increased pain. Ankle jerks absent. Diagnosis was made of brachial neuritis and sciatica. Bee venom therapy was begun, to which she responded promptly and was discharged on August 12, 1956. She has remained well to date.

CASE 27: M.L., a 50-year-old female, was seen on November, 1956, and gave a history of pain for ten years or more in the lower back, and in both knees and feet. Had pain also in the left knee. Some mornings she could not put the right foot on the floor without a cane. Walking made it worse. Examination disclosed acute pain in the right gluteal muscles, tenderness in the region of fourth, fifth and the first sacral vertebrae. Lasègue test was positive. Dorsiflexion increased the pain. The ankle jerks were absent. There was some rigidity in the lumbar spine and limited motion of the left knee. The diagnosis was osteoarthritis, confirmed by X-ray, and sciatica. Bee venom injections were given and the response was good. On March 30, 1957, she was discharged from treatment, and has remained well to date.

CASE 28: F.L., a 55-year-old male, was seen on August 18, 1956. He stated that for ten years he had had pain in his right shoulder joint. If he raised his right arm, he could not lower it, and vice versa. Getting worse. Examination disclosed a tender right shoulder joint with painful and limited motion. X-ray showed irregularities of the glenoid fossa. Diagnosis, osteoarthritis; bee venom was given. Patient responded quickly and he was discharged as completely recovered. He remained well to date.

CASE 29: I.O., a 73-year-old male, was seen in February, 1957, with a history of pain, limited motion, difficulty in walking, and inability to bend or turn. Must use a cane. He is in constant pain in both hips, both knees and both shoulders. Has had surgery and every other type of available medical care, without results. Examination confirms the above. X-ray shows markedly advanced old hypertrophic arthritis changes of both hips. The joint spaces are almost completely obliterated, and there is intense irregular sclerosis of the articular margins. There is an extensive linear calcification in the soft tissues, etc. It was explained to the patient how little hope we can hold out to him and we instituted bee venom therapy. The only reason this case is mentioned is because the very first treatment relieved the patient from all his pain in both shoulders. We are proceeding with the balance of the treatment. NOTE: After more than nine months of treatment his other symptoms did not improve. The patient asked to discontinue further treatments.

CASE 30: H.R., a 60-year-old male, was seen in October, 1955, with a history of pain in his back for 15 years. For the last four years he had had pain in his right knee and in the cervical, dorsal and lumbo-sacral areas. Examination elicited tender and painful locations in all the above areas, difficulty when bending, sitting or rising. X-ray showed osteoarthritis in the cervical, dorsal and lumbo-sacral vertebrae. The right knee showed only slight changes. A diagnosis was made of osteoarthritis and bee venom therapy started. Patient responded well. At the end of his first course, November 28, 1955, he felt well and asked to be discharged.

CASE 31: A.J., a 60-year-old male, was seen on February 4, 1958. He suffered severe pain in the right arm, shoulder and forearm for about three weeks. Had ACTH without results. Pain is constant but worse upon exercise or if work is attempted. Cannot raise that arm. Diagnosed as brachial neuralgia, he received three injections of bee venom on alternate days and reported himself as perfectly well. Has been well since.

CASE 32: D.L., a 72-year-old female, was seen in May, 1958, suffering very severe pains in her left arm while undergoing intensive treatment by another physician for an old and serious circulatory condition. All that was done for her did not relieve her pain. When the patient's condition finally improved, however, I recommended a bee venom ointment locally applied, providing the attending physician approved. He consented gladly and the ointment was applied according to my directions. The patient improved dramatically and promptly. After using the ointment for about three weeks, she was discharged and she had no further discomfort.

CASE 33: A.M., a 72-year-old female, was seen on September 3, 1958, with a history that one year ago she began with having one joint after another become inflamed until all joints were affected. She suffered intensely. Several physicians in her home town in Arizona did what they could, but her condition continued to deteriorate. The cortisone she received impaired her hearing. She decided to go to one of our best known institutions for relief and remained there for about four weeks. Refusing to take more cortisone, she was discharged without results. She next went to another well-known institution in the West, where she remained six weeks, but her condition constantly worsened. She now returned to her home town in Arizona. Not being able to remain there for any length of time due to her suffering, she decided to come to New York to seek relief.

A local physician sent her to me.

Examination disclosed an acutely ill patient with generalized rheumatoid arthritis. She was reduced to 90 pounds. Her temperature was 103°F. For nearly the entire year she had been bedridden. Could not do anything during that time, which included walking, sleeping, eating, standing or sitting. She could not raise or flex her joints. She had to be carried into my office. She was the sickest patient I have seen.

A cursory physical examination confirmed the diagnosis. I assured her that her condition was not hopeless. Bee venom injections were initiated and the patient responded most promptly. The pain left her completely within 24 hours and a few days later she was able to do most anything, including walking, sitting up and lying down, sleeping, eating. She was even able to go out marketing with her husband and helped to carry some of the packages home.

After completing the first series of injections, she was given a vacation from treatments on October 3, 1958, for four weeks.

She returned for the continuation of the treatments on October 27. After she had three more treatments and felt perfectly well, she met with an accident with a resulting fracture of the hip. This caused her to return to her home town for surgical care, with my full approval and cooperation. I have not heard from this patient since.

CASE 34: A.F., a 55-year-old male, saw me in July, 1957, stating that for four months he has had pain in his back, which has since spread to both knees, both thighs and both shoulders. Finally, it extended also to both hands and to his neck. At the time of his first visit, the pain was mostly in his hands, shoulders and knees. His neck was still painful and he could not turn his head. He received daily injections of bee venom for two weeks when he felt perfectly well and was discharged. This patient has remained free of symptoms since.

CASE 35: J.F.G., a 55-year-old male, was seen in May, 1958, suffering from pain in his right toe and left knee. The toe has troubled him for four years while the knee began to give him trouble only six months ago. Cortisone was of no avail. Physical examination confirmed the presence of osteoarthritis of both knee and toe. X-ray also confirmed this. He was placed on bee venom on May 5, 1958. On July 27, he was given a vacation from treatment. At that time he felt quite well. He returned for an inspection on October 14 to report that he felt perfectly well. No treatment was given him. He returned again on December 26, 1958, when he was discharged as perfectly well. He has returned several times since to report himself perfectly well, the last time being December 24, 1959.

CASE 36: M.G., a 40-year-old female, saw me in May, 1958 with a history of constant recurrences of pain in her left arm and shoulder which began four years ago. Examination disclosed tender areas in both locations of which patient complained. X-ray confirmed an osteoarthritis of the left shoulder joint with calcium deposits. She was placed on bee venom therapy on May 19, 1958. On June 20, she was given a vacation from treatment. She did not return for further treatment but reported on June 4, 1959, that she has been perfectly well since discontinuing the treatment.

CASE 37: J.J.M., a 65-year-old male, was seen with a history of pain running down the back of his right thigh and leg. The pain was severe and constant. Examination showed the presence of an old sciatica. He was put on bee venom therapy on August 6, 1958. On August 20, 1958, he was discharged as perfectly well and he has continued without symptoms since.

CASE 38: L.S., a 66-year-old female, came to see me upon the recommendation of a London, England, physician who took care of her while in that city. She gave a history that for 20 years, on and off, she suffered severe pain in both knees. An examination and X-ray confirmed an osteoarthritis of both knees. She was given bee venom therapy for the first time on September 18, 1958. On November 7, 1958, she was given a vacation from treatment. She did not return for further treatment but on January 2, 1959, she reported herself as perfectly well.

CASE 39: S.E., a 64-year-old female, came to see me and gave a history that for nine years she has suffered from pain and disability in both knees. She had great difficulty in walking. Cortisone was of no avail. Examination and X-ray confirmed an osteoarthritis of both knees. She was put on bee venom on October 4, 1958. On October 22, she was given a vacation from treatment and she felt very well at that time. She returned for further treatment on January 2, 1959. The injections were continued till February 14, 1959 when she was discharged. She has remained without symptoms since.

CASE 40: J.W., a 72-year-old physician, consulted me and he gave the history of suffering severe pain in the muscles of his shoulders, neck and back. The pain was so severe that he was obliged to discontinue his practice. He was placed on bee venom therapy on November 20, 1958. On January 27, 1959, he was discharged as free of all symptoms and he resumed his practice. The patient has continued free of symptoms to date.

* * * * *

I do not include the more recent of my cases who have been spectacularly helped, preferring to wait until we can be sure that they are benefited for a lasting period of time. As indicated by the foregoing case histories, there should be every assurance that these recent patients will follow the same pattern as the ones who were treated previously.

Since 1952, I have treated more than 100 patients with bee venom. Approximately half were lastingly benefited—i.e., relieved of all symptoms. As the reader can see, the duration of the disease does not have very much to do with whether or not bee venom will be effective—it is the *kind* of affliction and its progression. I have found that the people I cannot help are those whose disease has progressed to the point where the bones and joints are *fused.* Even so, in some cases, we can sometimes relieve them of pain for varying periods.

Another group on which bee venom has little lasting effect are those unfortunates who have become "cortisone addicts." In some people, cortisone can be just as addictive as morphine, if not more so. In these cases the entire body metabolism is disrupted, and the victim comes to depend upon cortisone in the same way as does the heroin addict. These cortisone addicts are pitiful for a physician to behold, for he knows his own profession has induced the dependency (in most cases, unwittingly) and that his profession has nothing which will offer them succor.

Quite recently (July, 1961) I saw once again the effects of cortisone addiction. The patient, a once beautiful woman of 40, had a history of many years' addiction to cortisone. In the beginning, the diagnosis was rheumatoid arthritis at quite an early age (about 27). Her husband took her to many clinics and physicians in a desperate attempt to gain relief for her suffering. However, each physician, thoroughly beguiled by the propaganda emanating from orthodox headquarters, treated her with cortisone or its "newer" derivatives—which were supposed not to induce the side effects of "pure" cortisone. (Cortisone addiction, itself, was not considered as serious until very recently, when the wrecked bodies and minds of the numerous addicts could no longer be ignored by the orthodoxy.)

This woman was "moon-faced" as a result of the swelling which prolonged administration of cortisone induces. Her whole body was bloated and she could barely get out of bed. She complained of horrible pains almost everywhere—with or without cortisone. Yet she suffered such agonies without it, that each doctor in turn administered it routinely. Twice, her physicians, becoming alarmed, had tried cortisone withdrawal. She became progressively worse, however; and on one such withdrawal, contracted tuberculosis, for which she was hospitalized.

Although her prognosis was practically hopeless, I undertook bee venom treatment in July, 1961, because a medical friend of mine insisted I take the case. The first few injections of bee venom produced an astounding effect. The patient stated that she had "never felt so good" during the last 13 years. Her husband stated, exuberantly, that he felt his wife could really withdraw from cortisone now as she never had been "withdrawal symptomless" before—she was now without pain and felt "wonderful."

However, in several weeks, her drug addiction manifested itself again. She was not cured: the demand for the drug had only been temporarily assuaged in some manner by the bee venom. Now she began to crave it again—in fact, *had* to have it. In cortisone addiction, the patient cannot take the so-called "cold turkey" treatment (abrupt withdrawal) which the heroin or morphine addict has to undergo when he is caught and jailed as a criminal.

I put her back on cortisone as a last resort. She is now away from New York City, but I have some faint hope that when she returns, I can wean her away from cortisone and reinstitute bee venom. And I hope this time we can save her.

I do hope also that my medical colleagues who are now finally being awakened to the dangers of cortisone therapy in the long-term treatment of arthritis, may profit from my experiences and from those who have now finally sounded the warning in medical journals and elsewhere.

CHAPTER V

WORK DONE IN AMERICA COMPARED WITH WORK DONE IN OTHER COUNTRIES

In this chapter I shall name other workers in the research field and I will add the names of a large number of clinicians, the groups who actually treat and care for the sick, and cite some of their published opinions upon the results of their work with bee venom. These investigations were carried on in the best-known research centers and hospitals; and the published reports appeared in the most respected medical journals of the respective countries.

Having read these reports, you will be in a better position to realize what an enormous amount of work, both research and clinical, this literature represents. You may be amazed, also, to discover that the United States is very far behind most medical research, in spite of all the medical propaganda which tells us we are the best fed, the best medically-cared-for country in the whole world.

Some of this material is technical, but I have simplified it for you as much as possible in the Glossary, to enable you to read the text understandingly.

Only a small percentage of the foreign reports have reached the physicians in this country and very little has been published here. This amounts to a suppression of the facts.

Let us begin with the Germans, encompass the Russians and then finally end with some favorable U.S. reports which have been ignored by the very organizations which claim they are seeking a cure for arthritis and are in the forefront of the battle.

We may find that for various reasons we are not in the forefront at all but are being caught flatfooted: embarrassed and hard pressed to give a rational excuse when other nations surpass us not only in medicine but in other phases of scientific development. Does anyone now remember Sputnik I and the consternation it caused? I feel we are in the same category in medicine, though as yet the situation is not as seemingly dramatic.

In 1953, Dr. Reinwand reported as follows: "In my 20 years' experience at the Julius Hospital in Wuerzburg [Germany], I have not once come across any therapeutic agent which showed better results in the countless rheumatic cases which have come to my attention as the B preparation of bee venom."

In 1954 Dr. Steigerwald, of Munich Hospital in Wessobrunn, stated: "Transposition of the vegetative reaction in chronic polyarthritis is very often the reason for its therapeutic results. Observations over a period of many years on extensive case material moreover convinced us that, among other existing possibilities, bee venom constitutes, in my opinion, the best possible therapeutic potentiality for all such transposition therapy."

And since this method of treatment has proved entirely safe in the past, there seems to be little reason to doubt that it cannot be equally safe in the future if, before commencing treatment, the attending physician will first make certain the patient is not allergic to bee venom injections. This should not be difficult to determine, and it could be done in the doctor's office within minutes. Such susceptibility, rare indeed, could be eliminated by special treatment.

Professor Wolfgang Weichardt, Wiesbaden, stated: "In bee venom we have, as is well known, a remedy which has already been used for a long time as a lay-medicine, above all, in use for rheumatic diseases. The successes achieved are confirmed by critical research workers, who have frequently tried to determine the causes for its effects."

Newer investigations were made by Reinert. According to this author, bee venom possesses, due to its chemical composition and its physicochemical behavior, the properties of a *Proteose* (a form of semiprotein) which is distinguished by its high amount of *tryptophan* (an amino acid of protein). Further experiments were undertaken by Chr. Tetsch and K. Wolff at the Pharmacological Institute in Berlin. They compared the bee venom with snake venom and they found that there exists an analogy between Crotalus (snake poison) and bee venom:

"In the employment of bee venom, we are undoubtedly dealing with an agent having a multiple effect upon the human organism. However, certain general information can be obtained by quantitatively conducted small [animal] experiments.

"We believe, therefore, to be entitled to the conclusion that the activations produced by bee venom are not directly produced by the substance itself, but indirectly by fissure-products which it has caused to originate in the body.

"By the interposition of the skin, the harmfulness of this highly different poison is largely eliminated and the formation of activating fissure-products is very much favored."

Dr. Siegfried Becker, of the First Medical University Clinic, Vienna, wrote: "In the year 1928 at the forty-third Balneologen Congress in Baden near Vienna, Dr. 'A' explained the modern bee venom therapy. The injectable preparation was used by Wasserbrenner in 1928 at the 'Wiener Poliklinic,' with satisfactory results. Loebel and Simo worked in the same Klinic on ambulatory cases; they also used the bee venom therapy with satisfactory results. Bee venom therapy was used on about two hundred cases of different forms of rheumatism and in most cases the result was satisfactory; in others, the results were hopeful.

"We observed one hundred and twenty cases and grouped them as follows:

Disease	Cases	Good Results	Part Results	No Results
Primary Chronic Polyarthritis				
Rheumatoids	28	16	9	3
Infectious Monoarthritis	20	15	3	2
Bechterew (Spondylitis)	5	4	0	1
Arthritis Deformans	10	4	2	4
Sciatica	14	12	0	2
Neuralgias	18	10	4	4
Polyalgias (Endocrine)	25	4	6	15

"In the description we outlined of the bee venom therapy, the greatest advantage is the very exact and flexible method of controlling the dosage. Its usefulness is proven through the remote possibility of danger, the avoidable general reactions, and the almost total absence of important reactions. In view of these facts and because of the undoubted success achieved even in the difficult cases, we consider ourselves entitled to recommend bee venom to the practitioner as a valuable weapon in the fight against rheumatism."

Otto Ludwig, Berlin, in an address made during the third Viennese medical week, May, 1941, reported on the possibilities of using bee venom in the treatment of rheumatic disorders, especially typical and atypical gout. We will quote him here in abbreviated form:

"First, bee venom is not a cure-all of rheumatism and gout. Anyone who does not take this into account will only reap failure. On the other hand, bee venom in injectable form cannot be replaced by any other remedy, according to my knowledge of the therapeutic program for combating rheumatism effectually, worked out at our institute in the course of fourteen years. We have been using it more and more since 1928, and I may say that the number of patients *not* receiving bee venom—at least in the last years—has been growing *less* and *less* in proportion to the total number.

"If, therefore, we have been using bee venom in the framework of our over-all therapeutic measures—since 1928—in the treatment of rheumatic and gout patients and on a scale, moreover, as shown in the table [omitted here] and if we have remained with this therapy for thirteen years, then the value of this remedy in combating rheumatism surely becomes apparent. . . ."

Comments on the treatment of rheumatism by F. Steigerwald and H. Maurer of the Hospital of the City of Munich in Wessobrunn: "After a critical survey of the present state in treating rheumatism, the authors report their own favorable experience in using bee venom, preparation B, therapeutically on about one hundred accurately observed patients with chronic polyarthritis. The cases coming for treatment were those in which one or several joints were affected with rheumatic arthritis and in which the feverish stage of an acute relapse had already been overcome in the usual way by means of general therapy. For the most part, the larger joints, especially subjected to mechanical strains, were involved.

"In over *fifty* per cent, this treatment brought about complete freedom from pain, together with restoration of mobility in the joints, so that supplementary physical therapy became possible."

The authors summarize as follows:

"Chronic rheumatism of the joints and particularly its primary chronic form unfortunately still represents a therapeutic problem for which no satisfactory solution has been found. While even today salicylic acid along with pyrazolon derivatives play an important role in the treatment of acute joint rheumatism, the changing reorientation of the vegetative reaction-situation most frequently leads to therapeutic success. Observations made over a period of years on a large number of patients have shown us that bee venom offers among all others, many possibilities and the greatest therapeutic field for much reorientation therapy."

Koehler, of the First Internal Department of Urban Hospital, Berlin, treated *polyarthritis, arthritis deformans* and *Bechterew's* disease with bee venom. She summed up her observations by stating that the remedy "favorably influenced all the symptoms in those conditions; the swelling and pain of the joints gradually subsided and their improved motility was very noticeable."

Loebel and Simo, at the First Medical University Clinic, Vienna, used bee venom in about 200 severe cases of primary and secondary chronic polyarthritis and obtained good results. It was found to be especially effective in myalgia and neuralgia cases. They thought that bee venom was worth further experiments.

Novotny, of the Orthopedic Hospital, Vienna, published in 1932 twenty cases of chronic inflammatory conditions which he had treated during the two preceding years with injectable bee venom. There were cases of amputations, in which ulcers developed in the stumps and they resisted all other known therapeutic measures. He injected bee venom intradermally over the infiltrated areas and found the results distinctly favorable.

Roch, of the medical faculty at Geneva, wrote an article in 1928 in which he expressed grave doubts about the claims of Terc and Keiter, almost doubting their published results. However, he said, that he had to take Professor Langer's word that "these men are no charlatans." In 1933, Roch showed an entirely different attitude, and he published 14 cases treated with bee venom:

10 cases of sciatica: 7 very good results; 3 fair results.
2 cases of lumbago: 2 very good results.
2 cases of chronic rheumatism: 2 improvements.

He continued to use bee venom and reported other cases with good results. Finally, he asked his assistant, Dr. M. A. DuBois, to give him a series of bee venom injections for what was diagnosed as osteoarthritis of the knee. The condition having been very obstinate, and since no relief was obtained despite all efforts, osteosarcoma (bone cancer) was suspected. Before he consented to an amputation, Dr. DuBois gave him the bee venom injections, with excellent results. The amputation was no longer necessary. Roch reported the entire episode to the Congress of Rheumatism in Paris.

Dr. Wolfgang Harter of the Rheumatism Institute, Vienna, wrote: "The principle of the bee venom lies in the fact that patients ailing with rheumatism of any type should be treated with the venom until they become immune to it.

"Certain concentrations of the venom make it most adaptable for treatment of nervous disorders. I had the opportunity to treat a larger number of patients with such disorders, after they were very carefully selected, and secured full cures, which were checked six months later for further confirmation.

"The cases treated with that concentration who were cured, and after six months showed no change in their conditions, are: *none.*"

J. Walch, of the University of Lausanne, wrote (abbreviated): "*Clinical Effects of Preparation B.* We treated about one hundred cases of rheumatic diseases; acute conditions like lumbago, myalgias, polyneuritis, sciatica (in cases of acute polyarthritis we did not use bee venom) and chronic diseases like chronic joint rheumatism, as well as chronic non-inflammatory joint diseases.

"End Result: After the observation of about one hundred cases treated with preparation B at the Lausanne polyclinic, we came to the conclusion that the preparation B of the bee venom is especially useful in the treatment of acute and sub-acute Myalgias, Epicondilitis, and especially in Periarthritis humero-scapularis [see Glossary for definitions]. Salicylic treatments and physiotherapy did not show any results. Furthermore, we achieved improvements in neuritis and polyneuritis and in sciatica. In arthritis and arthritics, bee venom, 'preparation B' was also used successfully."

The author of this article mentions in conclusion that "the results achieved with bee venom, preparation B, show real progress and bring to the patient only a minimum of danger."

Dr. B. Marinescu of the Neurological Clinic, Bucharest, wrote: "To recapitulate, we may say that from the summary presentation of eight of the more important cases drawn from a much greater number of different cases treated at our clinic, the beneficial effect of bee venom in treating rheumatic complications is manifest.

"Even though we do not as yet know exactly how this venom acts, nevertheless, the therapeutic effect of the bee venom in those cases of arthritis, myalgia, neuralgia, etc., in which we previously excluded syphilis, tuberculosis, and gonorrhea complications, emerges with certainty from our own experience as well as from that of others."

Maurice Perrin and Alain Cuenot, Nancy, France, addressed the Third International Congress on Rheumatism, Paris, France (paraphrased):

The authors reviewed the literature and gave various points in technique and then made the observations that "as a result of treatment with bee venom C, patients felt better, were less stiff, were more agile, and their entire body showed marked signs of improvement. These beneficial results have been obtained even with older people, in whom it works wonders."

The venom, they further stated, "has a tonic effect and all patients have benefited in their general conditions; they gained weight; their appetite improved; they slept better." "Altogether," they stated, "the tonic effect of the bee venom is absolutely remarkable. It is an anti-rheumatic remedy of the first order and we are already convinced of the good possibilities of bee venom as a treatment against rheumatism."

The authors presented the cases of 19 patients from their own practice, who were representative of the various types of rheumatism. They cited the history, symptoms, duration and treatment received by each of the patients, concluding with the results achieved in every case. These results were very satisfactory in nearly every instance.

In summing up, the authors stated, among other things, "The bee venom has important analgesic properties which are able to effect cures in some, and improve other type attacks of rheumatism which cause deformities, etc."

Dr. Rudolph Dimter, Vienna, of the Lainz Old People's Home for Incurables (abbreviated): "Only severe and very severe cases are admitted at our Institution. There was a certain amount of skepticism about any future success, the more so as we have had a great deal of previous disappointment with various other preparations. This time, however, we were agreeably surprised. Although—up to now—I have been urged by various doctors who worked with me to publish successful cases we had treated, but so far, I have always declined to do so. The reason was that I did not wish to give a report about temporary improvements, as the reputation of our Institute makes it necessary to observe a certain time limit before giving an opinion. This is especially important in cases of the slowly creeping Rheumatoid Arthritis, which forms the main contingent of all our cases. I would like to state here that, in the above-mentioned hopeless cases, it takes a lot of patience to render a progressive case stationary—one who has been bed-ridden for years, to walk again to a certain extent—sometimes even to make him fit to work again within limits. I would also like to mention here that, from our patients treated with bee venom A, we picked only cases where we did not rely merely on the subjective statements of the patients, but in order to avoid any suggestion induced by the wish for improvement, where we could check and rely upon the purely clinical report, that is, the actual function of the joints, to show us the failure or success of the treatment. In very recent cases, we took pictures at the start and during treatment and, by doing so, tried to create a documentary on moving films of the respective greatest possible movement of the diseased joint.

"We never were able to find any traces or signs of any virus in the bloodstream. We succeeded, however, with indirect findings with smears from tonsils and boils, and two months later, found indications in the scabs of a ringworm infection. From all those objects, we bred *Staphylococci sur. haemolyticus.* The blood level showed no abnormalities at this stage and the blood pictures showed no variations from the normal either.

"Results achieved by the treatment with bee venom A were successful above all expectations. It is unfortunate that only the movie camera can give the right impression of the effects of this treatment.

"The purpose of this paper has been to draw the attention of doctors to this treatment and to encourage them to try and check bee venom A and to give it the attention it so richly deserves."

Dr. Klemens Wasserbrenner, of the General Polyclinic of Vienna, wrote in 1928 (abbreviated):

"Our experiments with Apicosan [bee venom] have been conducted on 121 patients during one year. The following diseases were represented:

Sciatica	45 patients
Plexus neuralgia	16 patients
Intercostal neuralgia	25 patients
Primary chronic arthritis	25 patients
Arthritis deformans	10 patients

"In summing up we already can pronounce a judgement in favor of bee venom preparation and recommend it especially for cases of resistant Neuralgia. We will continue our experiments in this field and publish our results in detail."

Dr. M. Lenczner, Ambulatorio Medico Mussolini, Bucharest, expressed the following in 1936 (abbreviated):

"The bee venom therapy is a kind of *Reiztherapie* [stimulation treatment] which shows evidence of specific action on the rheumatic factor. We have used it in subacute and chronic cases only.

"Every case should be thoroughly studied. A positive Wassermann is a contraindication of Immenin treatment.

"In summing up we state that treatment with bee venom represents an extremely valuable therapy."

Dr. Arpad Lux, chief of the Clinic for Rheumatism in Vienna, wrote:

"The nature of this disease precludes in itself the possibility of roentgenologic proof of any improvement in the more or less altered skeletal structure. But the subjective relief was so unequivocal and the swift restoration of the capacity to work so apparent, even in cases with serious alterations, that we must admit that Immenin [bee venom] has an anti-inflammatory action.

"The combined treatment with bee venom and various physical methods, has been found to be extremely successful in all cases. On the other hand, all other medicaments have been excluded, during bee venom treatment."

Dr. G. Balderman, military surgeon, in the *Medizinische Klinik* (a weekly for general practitioners) wrote:

"In the bee venom we have a remedy, which when propertly applied, is the valuable agent in the fight against rheumatic diseases and the damage done by them to our national manpower."

Dr. Hans Novotny, assistant, from the Vienna Orthopedic Hospital (abbreviated):

"We believe that our experiences enable us to recommend a trial treatment with bee venom, in cases of chronic infiltrates of nonspecific nature, in particular in cases of troublesome stump infiltrates [rheumatic affliction of amputated limbs]."

Dr. Joseph Pick, from the Anatomical Institute of the Vienna University (abbreviated):

"It must be mentioned that bee venom is not a single substance, but rather a combination of different substances. Therefore, the action of bee venom should be considered as a manifold one. Certain findings, for which I could find no explanation, can be interpreted in this sense: thickening of the alveolar walls in the lungs, leucocytosis [white blood cell activity] in the blood and changes in the liver cells. In short, a series of questions has been raised, which can be answered only by future research."

Professor Dr. Meesmann, from the University Hospital for Eye Diseases, Kiel (abbreviated):

"Bee venom represents a valuable addition to the treatment of rheumatic iritis; absence of a secondary reaction makes it possible to diagnose with considerable certainty the true rheumatic cases. By continuing the treatment until the appearance of a secondary reaction, with following true immunity, we can often prevent or mitigate a relapse. A cure can be achieved only when the treatment is continued until the appearance of the protective effect. Because the immunity is not permanent, the treatment must be repeated every six months. According to Dirr and

Graeber the essential part of the protective effect is to be found in hypercholesterinemia, [high blood cholesterol] which develops only in certain kinds of rheumatic diseases and is of great importance both for differential diagnosis and for prognosis."

G.P. Zaitsev and V.T. Poryadin, Second Moscow State Medical Institute, U.S.S.R. (report published April, 1961, and translated from the Russian; abbreviated):

Experiments on the treatment of surgical disease with bee venom.

"During the past 2½ years at the clinic of general surgery of the Second Moscow State Medical Institute and in the three polyclinics of Moscow, 400 patients (ages 20-70) were treated with bee stings. The stings were found to be very effective in the following diseases: *Ankylous spondylosis deformans, spondylarthritis deformans, polyarthritis deformans, endoarthritis, atherosclerosis* of *peripheral vessels, thrombophlebitis,* tropical ulcers and slowly granulating wounds, *thyrotoxicosis.* In all cases, except ulcers and wounds, bee stings were first applied above the parathyroid glands and then at the affected place. Treatment lasted 30 days, with the stings (not more than 25) applied every other day. For ulcers and wounds the application was at 5 cm. from the edge of the affected place.

"There were no side effects, and in only three patients was an allergy noted. Reactions observed during the treatment were: increase in local temperature, normalization of sleep, appetite, stool: improvement in general well-being, increase in mental and physical tonus: decrease in weight of obese individuals, regularization of pulse and breathing; decrease in arterial pressure in hypertension. Out of the

150 patients with spondylarthritis and polyarthritis deformans, good results were obtained with 117, satisfactory results with 30, no change with 2; 1 was allergic. Out of 100 patients with endoarthritis and atherosclerosis of peripheral vessels, good results were obtained with 54, satisfactory results with 43, and no change with 3. Out of 50 patients with thrombophlebitis and varicose ulcers, results were good with 29, satisfactory with 19, and there was no change with 2. Biochemical studies of blood and urine were also carried out."

L.M. Shukhatovich, Polyclinic of the Fourth Moscow City Hospital, U.S.S.R. (April, 1961; abbreviated):

Applications of bee products in medical practice.

"The basic compound of bee venom is *mellitin,* which is very stable; it can be boiled or frozen without damage. Bee venom has bactericidal properties. Experiences in the clinics of the Soviet Union showed that bee venom exerts both general and local action on the human organism. It enlarges capillaries and small arteries, thus increasing the flow of blood to affected organs. Apitoxin [bee venom] has a beneficial effect on the viscosity and coagulability of blood, reduces the time of erythrocyte sedimentation [red blood cell separation] and increases general and local leucocytosis [white blood cell activity]. It exerts a stimulating effect on the heart muscle, lowers high blood pressure, and improves metabolism. Bee venom improves the general well-being of the sick, increases tonus and work ability, and improves sleep and appetite."

But lest you think no work has been done in the U.S., the following is taken from the *Annals of Internal Medicine,* January, 1938.

"Kroner and coworkers (1938), from the New York Hospital and the Department of Medicine of the Cornell University Medical College, treated 100 patients (25 males and 75 females) by intradermal injections of bee venom 'Apicosan,' a commercial product which contains the natural secretion of the honey bee in physiological saline solution. Many of the patients had previously undergone various forms of therapy without relief. The patients were divided into four groups: 1. Those with a markedly active and advanced form of arthritis with deformities present; 2. Those which present the typical picture of well-developed rheumatoid arthritis with characteristic peri-articular swelling of joints; 3. Those with severe pain of the joints but no swelling or deformities; 4. Those similar to group three but who had a corrected sedimentation rate within the normal range. The number of injections varied from six to 52 in a period of from one to 14 months. The patients who received a longer course of treatment showed a greater improvement on the average.

"Out of 100 patients, 73 showed improvement, of whom 35 showed marked improvement, and 38 showed moderate improvement. There was a definite and a lasting relief from the pain and swelling, and also a drop toward normal in the corrected sedimentation rate, if previously elevated. The highest percent of improvement occurred in the group of patients having a mild form of arthritis but with an elevated sedimentation rate. However, the patients with the same form of arthritis but with a normal sedimentation rate did not respond well to the treatment. This is probably due to the fact that many of the latter group were old or quiescent cases and some may not have had a true rheumatoid arthritis. This type of case does not respond well to any of the usual forms of therapy."

Kroner and coworkers concluded: "In estimating the results obtained from the study of an injectable form of bee venom ('Apicosan') for rheumatoid arthritis one is impressed with the definite improvement in the clinical symptoms and the significant drop in the corrected sedimentation index in the large percentage of patients. It would seem therefore that bee venom is worthy of further consideration." Oddly enough, Dr. Nichols, who later reported adversely on this study (Appendix G), was one of the coworkers in this experiment.

Dr. G. W. Ainlay of Nebraska treated 37 cases with "rapidly lyophilized bee venom solution" administering it intradermally. In 1939 the following results were published in the *Nebraska Medical Journal:* "Of these cases 11 were acute and 26 chronic. The patients were 26-67 years old (61 per cent were over 45 years old). Of these, 16 were completely cured; 16 had relief of pain, lessened swelling, nearly normal function; four were improved and had a considerable relief from pain, but there was little change in the swelling and deformities; one case was unaffected. This patient had a parathyroid disturbance with muscle spasms and bony deformities."

* * * * *

In the Appendix we deal with the so-called "negative" reports in our country and we will see why, in still another instance, our U.S. medicine, controlled by bureaucratic, authoritarian organizations, is not giving our people the medical care they deserve. For these bureaucrats in high places are primarily politicians having arrived at their exalted positions via their ability to administrate and control their colleagues rather than by exact scientific procedures.

Now that you have seen some of the evidence from my own patients and also a little of the monumental evidence which has been accumulated abroad, would you not think that those in control of American medicine would be forced to act? Would you think they could calmly and blithely ignore *all* the evidence for bee venom and even invent falsehoods about it? (See Chapter 7.)

I am sorry to report this is the case not only with bee venom, but with scores of other advanced treatments for many diseases. (For instance, the use of ultra-sound, with which President Kennedy was recently treated, has been employed for a decade or more in Europe and was, until fairly recently, roundly denounced by the "authorities" here as being a fake, or at least an ineffective remedy. The same with BCG, the antituberculosis vaccine, which for 30 years has been employed with success in Europe and now is only beginning to be recognized here. We could mention many other treatments which have been accorded short shrift in the U.S. and now have been acknowledged grudgingly by the medical powers only after great pressure engendered by their success abroad.

The problem is: can we afford the luxury of maintaining a medical hierarchy in our country which is so shortsighted, so bigoted in its own nonscientific opinions, that it will lag behind the rest of the world in treating its citizenry?

I am sorry that I had to write this book. Had bee venom been thoroughly investigated—as in foreign countries—my book would not have been necessary. I would not have had to appeal to the public or to the average doctor, which I am now frankly and unashamedly doing. I thank God that at least I have this final appeal and that we live in a country where some freedom of publication is possible, and that we have some recourse to the people—and to our colleagues.

Unfortunately, the truth is not always easy to disseminate, even medical truths—which, cursorily, would seem to be the easiest of all—since the medical spirit of inquiry asks, first of all: Does the proposed remedy, or procedure, work? If it does work in a significant number of cases, as reported by reliable investigators from all over the world (as in the case of bee venom), then the medical profession should accept these reports and begin using the therapy at once. The leaders of the medical profession should remember that the first duty of the physician is to his patient.

CHAPTER VI

WHAT ARE THE DANGERS OF CORTISONE?

Hormone steroids—cortisone and similar hormones—are substances secreted normally in small quantities by the adrenal and pituitary glands. The products now in use are not the natural secretions of those glands but the synthetic substitutes of the natural, recently developed. This makes it possible to produce them in huge quantities by mass production methods.

Now let us see why they have been so celebrated by the medical profession and why they are now falling out of favor.

In 1952, soon after the hormone steroids came into use, the A.M.A. held its convention in the city of Chicago. The head of the medical department of the Armour Laboratories, Chicago, Illinois, addressed the convention on a study their medical department had made upon the first 4,000 cases which had been treated with the product made by them, ACTH. The facts were furnished to the Armour medical department by 40 collaborating investigators in various parts of the country.

This was indeed the first study on that subject. The

results showed a large variety of complications, or so-called side effects, the existence of which caused consternation among the hearers. Some of these complications ran as high as 44 per cent, all the way down to less than 1 per cent. The complications included mental changes, edema, hypertension, heart failure, potassium deficiency, spontaneous infections, impaired wound healing, diabetes, peptic ulcers, hypothyroidism, thrombophlebitis, moon faces, "buffalo hump," menstrual irregularities, osteoporosis, and many others.

In addition to the complications, or side effects, there were 35 fatalities of patients who "died of causes felt by the investigators to be directly attributable to the side effects of ACTH."

No wonder there was consternation. Arthritis and rheumatism were not as a rule fatal diseases before the advent of these drugs. There was, however, a ready answer from those who were interested in the use by the medical profession of hormone steroids. The profession was advised to go right on using the drugs, but to reduce the size of the dosage. It was claimed that when this was done, improvement of the situation would follow. Physicians were also advised to observe more carefully the reactions of each patient, in order to prevent the complications. Nothing was said about the fact that the complications developed just as much in patients under the care of the best-trained specialists, as they did in the small country places where the very busy physician sometimes did not even have hospital facilities for such careful watching.

At any rate, the profession was put on the alert and cautioned about the dangers involved.

Now we come to 1956, four years later, when we had a

right to expect improvement in the situation. And here is what we found:

The situation was much worse. Not only because more sufferers were treated with the drugs, but also because the complications from them were cumulative and more had developed, in the intervening four years, among the old patients.

For these statements we have the authority of a report made by the special committee of the American Rheumatism Association, under the chairmanship of William D. Robinson, M.D., F.A.C.P., the University of Michigan, chairman, Editorial Committee.

This report was published in *Annals of Internal Medicine,* issued monthly by the American College of Physicians. The report took up about 250 pages, and covered a study of the American and English literature on arthritis and rheumatism—for the three most recent years only.

It is needless to say that we can mention only a very few portions of that report, since this entire volume would not be sufficient to cover the report adequately. The original is, of course, available in full.

"Untoward Effects: Much attention was devoted to the undesirable effects which develop during treatment with corticotropin or corticosteroids. The frequency of such undesirable effects varied in different series from 23% to 65%; and they were seen to some extent in 83% of 36 essentially normal young men treated with substantial amounts of ACTH or cortisone for 31 consecutive days. Determining factors appeared to be dosage, duration of treatment, individual susceptibility, and nature of the disease treated.

"Many of the untoward effects were attributable to the physiologic results of hyperadrenalism [overactivity of the adrenal gland]. These included the well recognized somatic changes of Cushing's syndrome, such as obesity, moon face, "buffalo hump," supra-clavicular fat pads, hirsutism and acne. Sodium retention accounted for fluid retention and presumably for cardiac enlargement and congestive cardiac failure.

"Osteoporosis: The frequency of osteoporosis, often with spontaneous fracture, cannot be estimated from several case reports. It occurred in three of 66 patients receiving ACTH or cortisone for a variety of diseases, nearly all being treated for six months or less. In another series of 56 patients, 7.1% developed osteoporosis. Women and older patients were more likely to develop this complication. . . .

"Psychologic and Central Nervous System Disturbances: Psychic disturbances, ranging from exaggerated degrees of the usual euphoria to severe psychoses of various types, occurred with sufficient frequency to constitute a real hazard in therapy. In several series of patients the frequency of distinctly aberrant psychologic reactions was 5.5% of 128 patients, 6.3% of 63 patients, and 15% of 66 and of 80 patients, respectively. Most of the psychoses were mild, transient and self-limited when the hormones were withdrawn but some required shock therapy, and suicides were reported. . . .

"Another serious complication was the development of convulsions, with or without accompanying psychosis. In two fatal cases, autopsy revealed no pathologic changes sufficient to account for the convulsions and coma. . . .

"Peptic Ulcer: There were numerous reports of activation of gastric or duodenal ulcers during cortisone or corticotropin therapy. In some cases there was no previous ulcer history. The ulceration was often first manifested as a complication, such as perforation or hemorrhage. Of

18 cases reviewed from the literature, 12 manifested perforation, hemorrhage, or both; there were 5 deaths from complications from peptic ulcer. Gastro-intestinal bleeding also occurred in the absence of lesions demonstrable by X-ray. . . .

"Activation or spread of tuberculosis was of special concern. The development of tuberculous meningitis and of miliary tuberculosis during or closely following the use of corticotropin or cortisone was recorded. The activation of pulmonary tuberculosis in patients receiving these hormones for rheumatoid arthritis was described repeatedly. Other infections included pneumonia, purulent pericarditis, peritonitis, and abscesses at the site of intramuscular injection.

"Toxic Reactions to Phenylbutazone: The incidence of toxic reactions was high. In the largest series—800 patients —40% developed some evidence of toxicity; this was severe enough to require discontinuation of the drug in 15% of the 800. Review of the literature prior to June, 1953, yielded an average 22% of 1,526 patients who experienced toxic reactions. Eleven deaths attributed to this drug were briefly noted. . . .

"Edema was attributable to sodium retention. It occurred in 14% of patients in two large series and was noted by most workers. This effect presumably was responsible for occasional cases of hypertension, pulmonary edema and congestive heart failure. Other cardiac complications included tachycardia, arrythmias and myocardial infarction. [See Glossary for definition.]

"The serious toxic potentialities of phenylbutazone posed a real problem regarding its use. 'Although the patient may often be prepared to take any risk for relief of symptoms, his physician usually is not! In a symposium of the Empire Rheumatism Council it was concluded that, although anti-rheumatic action is hard to define, the action of phenylbutazone in this regard has not been convincingly established and there has been no suggestion of a curative action.' In these circumstances, phenylbutazone should not be used merely as an alternative analgesic in rheumatism. Careful selection of patients and close attention to signs of toxicity are now rightly demanded. . . .

"Results of Therapy: There was general agreement that corticosteroids and corticotropin therapy is only suppressive and does not result in lasting remissions. Maintenance cortisone therapy was found beneficial for some, but not practical for all patients. . . .

"Conclusions Regarding Corticosteroids and Corticotropin: The literature covered in this Review reflects a period in which the limitations and dangers of therapy with these agents became sharply defined. As these facts became more widely appreciated, the high hopes held for these agents as a panacea for rheumatoid arthritis gave way to disillusionment in some quarters. The opinion that these hormones yielded no better long-range results than conventional methods of treatment was supported by one study, in which the status of 27 patients who had received moderate doses of cortisone for one to three years was not clearly superior to retrospective but carefully matched control cases. Some felt that the patients with rheumatoid arthritis were probably not getting as good care as before cortisone. . . ."

Thus the second phase of the these so-called wonder drugs came to an end. Their value in therapy for arthritis and rheumatism, which always require treatment for prolonged periods, were almost completely discredited.

No wonder that, on February 2, 1957, the New York

World Telegram and Sun printed an interview with Dr. Russell L. Cecil, Medical Director of the Arthritis and Rheumatism Foundation, in which he is quoted as stating:

"Cortisone is being used in less than 20% of cases, and ACTH is being used even less. Why? One answer is the unfavorable side effects. These have included moonlike rounding of the face, growth of hair, skin troubles, muscular weakness, retention of fluids, and emotional instability."

Hence, it became imperative to begin to talk about newer and better drugs. If they were not really newer or better did not matter much. Madison Avenue would attend to the problem of selling them to the public; and Madison Avenue did just that.

So now we come to the latest posture—and the funniest —of the hormone steroids, and the sales flip-flop to put over these products in a different guise; in the name of research and all for public good, of course.

Madison Avenue laid plans for a huge celebration in the form of a Conference, run under the title of:

CONFERENCE

on

A DECADE OF ANTI-INFLAMMATORY STEROIDS

FROM CORTISONE TO DEXAMETHASONE

Monday, December 15 and

Tuesday, December 16, 1958

All Sessions will be held at

The Barbizon-Plaza Hotel

101 West 58th Street at 6th Avenue

New York 19, New York

The following three organizations participated in the running of the Conference: the New York Academy of Sciences, Merck, Sharp & Dohme Research Laboratories and Schering Corporation.

To this celebration was invited a group of special guests, many of whom were prepared to read papers on the wonders of the very latest hormone steroids. They came from England, Canada and from all over the United States. The stage was set for an enthusiastic welcome to the new brainchild of Madison Avenue. Advance bulletins were distributed lauding this new steroid "dexamethasone" as the last word in research, upon which no expense was spared to make it perfect.

The author must have been invited through some error.

A number of papers were read. I will now quote from some of those papers, all by friends of the last word in scientific research. Yet, even while the celebration was going on, it is interesting to note what some of the authors of the papers allowed themselves to say:

Edward W. Boland, M.D., of Los Angeles, California, said, among other things, "The over-all incidence of adverse reactions from dexamethasone (Decadron) was about the same as from prednisolone [a form of hydrocortisone] when equally effective antirheumatic doses were given. . . . Dexamethasone appeared to have about the same tendency as prednisolone to provoke facial mooning, supraclavicular fat pads [buffalo hump], and hypertrichosis [abnormal hair growth] when the drugs were given in doses of corresponding anti-rheumatic strength.

"The rate of occurrence (56%) and the severity of ecchymatic skin lesions [purple skin blotches] with dexamethasone were greater than with prednisolone.

"Among the most common side effects encountered, and certainly the ones that were most objectionable to patients, were quickening of appetite (30% of cases), excessive weight gain (23%), and the development of abdominal girth (17%).

"Approximately 10% of the patients experienced abdominal distention or bloating. In two instances this was so pronounced that treatment was changed to another steroid.

"Clinical experience with the compound has not been sufficiently long, however, to warrant a final appraisal of its over-all therapeutic efficiency—that is, its capacity to maintain suppression of disease activity in relation to the avoidance of objectionable side effects."

Oswald Savage, M.D., of the West London Hospital, London, England, read a paper in which he said, among other things:

"Difficulties occurred with these long term cases when conditions requiring surgery arose. In the ordinary run of life, with a group of patients who have been restored to independence and are working, some will inevitably meet with accidents and with incidents such as strangulated hernia, appendicitis, and sepsis.

"Surgeons in our country were reluctant to operate on patients using steroids because they feared the wounds would not heal. Often, without our knowledge they would stop the drug, not realizing that they were running a real risk of post-operative adrenal crises. [Adrenal failure is a result of the long-term steroid therapy.] It has been an uphill struggle to educate our surgeons in this matter.

"There is no particular advantage in having a stronger

steroid for, to the patient, it is just another tablet to be taken through the day and, for the physician, minor adjustments of dosage are more difficult.

"These trials, including large groups of patients with varying degrees of rheumatoid activity, showed no difference between cortisone and salicylates [which are, as almost everyone knows, "aspirin"]. They did not show, nor were they designed to show, what is needed for a particular patient, with severe rheumatoid arthritis who, despite all efforts of the physician, is rapidly becoming crippled."

In discussing this paper, Charles Slocum, M.D. (University of Minnesota, Mayo Foundation and Mayo Clinic, Rochester, Minn.), said: "I think that we have all seen a considerable number of undesirable effects, and I cannot be quite as optimistic about the relative safety of accepting them as has been suggested."

B. Rose, M.D., of the McGill University Clinic and the division of allergy, Royal Victoria Hospital, Montreal, Canada, read a paper and said in part:

"However, reports have appeared that expressed a considerable divergence of opinion concerning the basic value and potential dangers of the steroids. Thus, some appear to use them with little fear of undesirable effects, whereas others have condemned them almost without reserve. Such variations of opinions are understandable when it is recognized that their basic mechanism of action is still obscure, that symptoms will usually recur after the drugs are withdrawn, and that continued use may lead to a variety of undesirable effects, some of which may be fatal.

"All other undesirable effects such as mooning of the face, hirsutism, osteoporosis, and impairment of carbohydrate tolerance can and do occur with the newer compounds. . . .

"The suppression of both the pituitary as well as adrenal function by long-term steroid therapy has been emphasized by others; pertinent to this are the findings of Burrage and co-workers, who observed morphologic [cellular change] signs of atrophy of both adrenals and pituitary at autopsy of patients who had been on long-term steroid therapy. . . .

"Since it is not possible to determine in which patients the pituitary adrenal axis has been suppressed, it has been our practice to regard all individuals who have received steroid therapy as potential cases of adrenal insufficiency and to treat them accordingly in stressful situations. . . .

"However, it is to be emphasized that the abandonment of all orthodox methods of treatment in favor of the easy use of steroids for the control of allergic disease cannot be condemned too strongly. A large percentage of patients with allergy can be managed without benefit of steroids.

"Finally, it should be pointed out that anti-inflammatory steroids are useful and acceptable means of treatment in patients who have failed to respond to all other forms of therapy. It is clear, furthermore, that judicious management, keeping the dose as low as is compatible with freedom from symptoms, and the use of adjunct forms of therapy have permitted many chronic invalids to return to a useful way of life. To give a patient anti-inflammatory steroids without advising him of the nature of the compound, and without adequate and frequent follow-up is to do him an injustice that may lead to serious consequences."

J.D.H. Slater and co-workers report on dexamethasone,

the latest and supposedly the best steroid, in an article published in the *Lancet,* London, 1:173-177, Jan. 24, 1959, which they conclude with the following:

"The adrenal-suppressing and diabetogenic [diabetes-inducing] effects are comparable to those of the older steroids. Metabolic studies suggest that undesirable side-effects are likely in some patients and at this stage there is no justification for any claims about freedom from side-effects. . . ."

The *British Medical Journal* (1:109-110, Jan. 10, 1959), had an editorial on "A Decade of Anti-Inflammatory Steroids" in which it states in part:

"Cortisone might still be the steroid of choice if it were not for its side effects. In large dosage it causes salt and water retention as well as a diabetic state, and may induce edema and hypertension. Because of its catabolic effect it may cause osteoporosis and pathologic fractures of vertebrae. Fluorohydrocortisone, because of its marked sodium-retaining action, is valueless as an anti-inflammatory substance except in the topical therapy of skin diseases. . . .

"While prednisone and prednisolone have lower sodium-retaining action than cortisone, they tend more to produce peptic ulcers which are often asymptomatic until they bleed or perforate. . . .

"It is perhaps too soon to assess its liability to produce side-effects. There is some evidence that it causes less disturbance of carbohydrate metabolism, but it may induce weight gain, mooning of the face, and abdominal distention. . . ."

But if more proof of the dangers of cortisone were

needed, it was adequately provided on June 22, 1961, when Dr. Cornelius Traeger, assistant clinical professor of medicine at Cornell Medical School told the American Rheumatism Association that some of his patients were doomed because they were addicted to cortisone and could not be "weaned."

Dr. Traeger said: "Fortunately, not all patients become addicts. But we must be wary when we use cortisone or similar drugs. It's the treatment of last resort, *after all else fails.*"

In his eleven cortisone addicts, Dr. Traeger noted such toxic effects as heart pain, stomach ulcers, high blood pressure, destruction of the bone joints, osteoporosis (fragile bones) and purple skin patches.

Dr. Traeger's observations on cortisone addicts have now been corroborated by many researchers, including the author, who first noticed this phenomenon several years ago before publication was possible.

So now, we have fatalities from the use of hormone steroids; we have a new set of diseases among those who have received this therapy. While we are apparently relieving pain temporarily in some cases, those patients, and others, are convicted to lifelong medical care. We cause excessive hair growths on the faces and other parts of many women. We create new patients all the time. In many cases, the continued employment of the steroid hormones spreads the disease and makes the condition permanent. The adrenal gland becomes atrophied, which is also true of other vital organs. When the physician advises patients to discontinue treatments because of side effects like hypertension, ulcers, hemorrhage, diabetes, psychological disorders, etc., the patients find themselves physically, morally, and intellectually depressed, so that some envision suicide. It is also true that in many cases, when treatment with the steroid hormones is discontinued, patients find themselves so stiff and unable to move, that they are forced to remain addicted to the therapy.

Bee venom stimulates the production of cortisone and ACTH in the body. This, however, we must understand, is done in harmony with the other known 31 hormones produced in the adrenal gland in the way and in quantities needed in the human body for normal functions. Finally, we must remember that the steroid hormones employed are not the genuine product and, apparently, a poorly synthesized imitation of it. This imitation tends to create a glandular imbalance.

So we have fatalities, many types of complications and so-called side effects, from the use of the steroid hormones.

What a high price we are paying for so little!

Again I ask, *What is there to celebrate?*

The new products are not better than the old, and sometimes they are even worse. No matter how much improvement has been tried over the past years—even when the picture improved slightly in some respects—the new drugs came out worse than the old ones in other respects, with new and more dangerous side effects.

Physicians reading the advertising put out by the pharmaceutical houses do not recognize the products for what they really are. Yet most physicians depend for their medical reading upon the journals which publicize these less than half truths.

We are not dealing here with a purely scientific research effort, but with a persistent attempt to make the steroid hormones fit into a picture where they cannot ever fit because of the grave dangers involved with treatment for prolonged periods, as is the case with arthritis and rheumatism.

It is high time to look into other methods. Methods of proven effectiveness in many cases, devoid of dangers when properly employed, and which can be used by every general practitioner no matter where located.

Only through the employment of a method every general practitioner can have at his disposal can we hope to help the many millions who so urgently need that help.

CHAPTER VII

MY FIGHT FOR BEE VENOM RECOGNITION

As pointed out in the other chapters, certain powerful forces in official medical circles are hindering the spread of knowledge about bee venom as a treatment for arthritis and rheumatism. Two principal agents in the fight against the acceptance of bee venom as a legitimate treatment are the drug firms, which discover, promote, and sell steroids, and the leaders of the medical profession, who choose to remain slaves to steroid treatment. A third contributing element is the strength of old, outmoded fabrications that linger on in the memory of some physicians, even prominent ones.

From a purely material standpoint, the pharmaceutical industry in this country has a great deal to gain from large-scale production of the various corticosteroids. Bee venom costs much less than the latest steroid hormones; and the drug companies realize that fully. By making bee venom scarce, they force the doctor to use the steroid treatment for arthritis and rheumatism. In this case they have a conflict of interests. While they exist to serve the medical profession by making available the best of drugs and medications, they are also dedicated to profit from their efforts.

As recent committee investigations show in detail, the companies continue to promote extensively their new drugs, without regard to their real efficacy. They boldly claim all sorts of good to accrue from their products, but in small print they add, as a precaution, that a still better remedy is in the offing. Thus the public is encouraged to believe they have the best of medication when they may actually have an intermediate, and possibly unsuccessful, remedy.

Much more responsible than the drug companies are the so-called leaders of the medical profession, for they hold the reins of research. They are slaves to steroids. Because they lack courage to free themselves, they have jeopardized our chance to progress.

The blame must be laid at their feet for having so long ignored the flood of literature from Europe on bee venom and its power in healing arthritis and rheumatism. As much as the public, and possibly more, doctors need education regarding this therapy.

Acceptance of a false belief can do irreparable harm to one afflicted with arthritis. If he chooses the wrong method of treatment, he will suffer with no chance of permanent relief, of being restored to health and a useful life. If apathy and doubt crowd out hope, he can forfeit effective permanent relief. The responsibility of medical leaders is to handle the problem of these two crippling diseases with courage and foresight.

The strength of hand-me-down tales of bee stings and their effects on rheumatism and arthritis sufferers lingers on, cropping up occasionally in the opinions of prominent physicians. This tendency of outmoded opinion to rule modern science is illustrated by the following incident.

About three years ago, an eminent physician with an international reputation, Dr. Walter C. Alvarez, wrote in his syndicated newspaper column that bee venom was useless for the treatment of rheumatism and arthritis. The entire article was based, not on recent research, but on his experience of 50 years ago.

About the turn of the century, the daily press reported on a severely afflicted arthritic who, after being attacked by a swarm of bees and painfully stung, had recovered the use of his joints. Since physicians believed at that time that formic acid was the chief ingredient of bee venom, some began to inject the acid around the joints of their arthritis and rheumatism patients. None recovered and the doctors, soon discouraged by their efforts, wrongly declared that bee venom had no curative powers.

Actually, they had proved that *formic acid* had no such ability. But 50 years later, our friend was willing to write a column based completely on his experience as a *young intern* who had also tried formic acid. He even seemed unaware that research had established that formic acid is not even an ingredient of the bee poison.

After reading the article, I wrote a letter to Dr. Alvarez on November 25, 1958, in which I stated:

> . . . If you still believe what you wrote 3 years ago, I would like to explain that the reason your 50 patients did not get well, or did not get any benefit from the formic acid injections, is because there is *no* formic acid in bee venom.
>
> It is perfectly true that 50 years ago it was believed that formic acid was an important constituent of the venom. However, the work of a number of research workers since that time

proves that formic acid is not at all a constituent of bee venom.

Should you wish to look further into the subject, I respectfully refer to you the work of . . . . [about a dozen references were cited]. Finally, I take the liberty to quote from the above cited work of Forster [Karl August Forster; reference not reprinted here] in which he sums up the subject:

"Summarizing, it can now be said that there is no further doubt that in dealing with the effective portion of bee venom, we are dealing with a protein-like substance."

Not having heard from you in a long time, I hope that this will find you in good health, and thanking you for past courtesies,

Sincerely yours,
JOSEPH BROADMAN, M.D.

To this I received a reply dated December 1, 1958, reading:

DEAR DR. BROADMAN:

Thank you for your letter. Yes, several people called my attention to my mistake. . . .

Cordially,
WALTER ALVAREZ, M.D.

Although the physician frankly admitted his mistake to me in a private letter, he did not make a public retraction, to the best of my knowledge. Instead, he compounded the error by attacking bee venom again in 1961, in virtually the same language he had used previously! It is almost inconceivable to me how a physician of his standing can apologize privately to me, admitting his "mistake," and then later repeat the same mistake in public print. He owes it to his readers and to the public in general to rectify an error that he has helped to perpetuate. By writing these two misleading articles, he has undoubtedly renewed many physicians' hostility to the most effective treatment known today for arthritis and rheumatism.

By way of comparison, Dr. Herman N. Bundesen (now deceased) was also an eminent physician with an international reputation. Among his many public and civic activities, Dr. Bundesen also contributed a syndicated medical column to some of the country's best newspapers. On December 31, 1958, he, too, wrote an article for his papers on the subject of bee venom. Here is what he wrote:

"BEE STING MAY RELIEVE RHEUMATISM. . . .

"About 11,000,000 Americans suffer from arthritis, rheumatism or one of the other rheumatic diseases.

"Chances are overwhelming that not a single one of them is a beekeeper!

"Now you may snicker at this fact, but it has real medical significance. For centuries the general public has attributed the virtual immunity of beekeepers from arthritis and rheumatism to the repeated stings of bees.

"Ancient physicians, and even some during much more recent times, believed that the stings of bees helped prevent arthritis and rheumatism and helped cure them after they had developed.

"Apparently their patients complained of the technique, however, for treating persons with bee stings isn't practiced any more. At least I hope it isn't!

"Yet the beneficial factor of the bee sting is readily available. Not only has bee venom been isolated and purified, it even has been standardized.

"Dr. Joseph Broadman, who has made quite a study of the value of bee venom in treating rheumatism and arthritis, reported in a recent issue of *General Practice* that tens of thousands of persons have been treated with this method without any side effects, complications or fatalities.

"He says those who have had experience with bee venom praise it very highly. And he says that use of bee venom in such cases 'merits the careful consideration of the general practitioner.'

"Now Dr. Broadman, who has had scientific papers published by numerous medical journals, doesn't claim that this form of treatment will cure all patients. However, he does feel that bee venom will give 'large numbers' of rheumatic and arthritic patients 'substantial relief.'

"Many early cases, he adds, will obtain permanent relief, although others will get only partial results. Some, of course, will get no benefit at all.

"The simplicity of the use of bee venom, Dr. Broadman says, 'lends itself to the practice of general practitioners everywhere.' "

With the aid of a few others, I have tried to spread knowledge of the advantages of bee venom treatments for sufferers from arthritic and rheumatic diseases. To gain the meager success achieved so far has required extreme effort.

I managed to achieve publication in only one medical journal in the United States (*General Practice,* see Appendix). Then all avenues closed for future articles on bee venom. The first article was mailed to nearly every medical journal in the country. Two or three responded favorably, but did not publish the article. One journal accepted, only to return the article to me near publication time. The explanation: two members of the editorial committee, who were especially interested in arthritis and rheumatism, "objected" to its publication.

Another journal's editor wrote me, stating the article would be considered for publication if revised in accordance with certain specifications. I gladly agreed to rewrite the article and when submitted, it was promptly accepted. But when the article reached the executive office, I received a letter (in October, 1957) informing me that the article would be published in early 1958. More than four years have passed and the article has not been published and my correspondence has been ignored.

While on the subject of rejection slips, let me list another one. I sent an article to a medical journal with a national circulation emphasizing that any general practitioner could treat patients suffering from arthritis or rheumatism with bee venom and could secure far better results (not exposing his patients to the dangers of side effects and complications, for example) than with the steroids now in use. The publication had asked its readers to contribute articles which might interest or help other physicians or their patients.

Since I thought it a good opportunity to publicize vital information not available in most medical journals, I prepared a special article in which, after stating the facts as persuasively as possible, I presented a bibliography of no less than 85 articles (on the subject of bee venom) written by well-known authorities in Europe and in America. All related some experiences with the treatment for all forms of arthritis and rheumatism. Surely, I reasoned, so important an array of confirmation and proof would move the editors into accepting the article.

I was wrong. With the explanation "it doesn't quite

meet our needs," my manuscript was returned. Their needs could be easily seen from the journal's contents, which dealt mainly with economic problems relating to the practice of medicine. Its entire income seems to come from page after page of pharmaceutical advertising.

Here we can see another possible reason for the difficulties I have encountered. A publisher of a medical journal does not like to print material to which his advertisers may object, or which recommends medical remedies not prominently advertised. If those advertised products were as good as hoped, this sensitivity might be excused. But the steroids (to be specific) are not beneficial for arthritic and rheumatic sufferers.

What is the physician's usual answer to the patient who asks about bee venom as a method of treatment for his arthritic or rheumatic condition? Let's follow a friend of an arthritic patient of mine. Having heard that his friend has obtained relief from me through bee venom, he decides to talk the matter over with his own physician. The doctor's stock answer goes something like this:

"Mr. H, like many arthritic patients, you have been coming here for some time. From the very beginning I have been telling you that nothing more can be done than is being done here. I have told the same to other patients, and other doctors have been consulted to confirm my opinion. If there's any good in the bee venom treatment, I must confess skepticism and a certain amount of ignorance regarding its value."

And what the doctor does not know is that hundreds of doctors abroad have used bee venom in the successful treatment of tens of thousands of patients without one serious complication, side effects, or fatality. I have had the same results with many of my patients who have been relieved of suffering and, in many other cases, completely cured. Patients are cured within three weeks, sometimes within six months. In extreme cases treatment may last an entire year or even more. Often I can only arrest pain or give a partial result. I make no fantastic claims. Yet many patients have come to me after years of treatment from other doctors and, while skeptical of new methods, were overjoyed to learn that they could lead normal, healthy lives in place of ones filled with pain and frustration.

I have earned many enemies and few friends precisely because I insist on clarifying the most efficient and beneficial methods of treatment for rheumatism and arthritis. There are many people, however, who do not want the truth preserved. Education to them is a farce. In creating the Broadman Library on War, Peace and International Relations I did not seek praise, but only the preservation of truth for future generations. Even in that work some criticized me for not devoting my full time to the practice of medicine. In the same way, others oppose truth in medical science.

CHAPTER VIII

WHAT YOU CAN DO

Conclusions drawn in preceding chapters may now be summarized as:

1. It is my considered opinion that bee venom is a specific for arthritis and rheumatism. No steroid hormone even claims to be such.

2. Once it has been determined that no allergy against the substance is present, there is practically no further danger entailed in the treatment. The administration of this treatment usually runs a smooth course and often brings many pleasant surprises to both patient and physician.

3. The only types of rheumatic cases bee venom does not affect favorably with any degree of promptness are the very old, the very chronic, the very feeble, and those addicted to cortisone. It can hardly be expected that such cases can be cured by any possible new discovery. Nothing can repair such terrible neglect or misfortune.

From the foregoing, it is evident that in bee venom we have an effective treatment with which to fight arthritis and rheumatism. What is needed now is a large-scale, educational effort to bring to each physician knowledge of the most recent techniques. The health of millions of Americans suffering from rheumatism in any form is at stake. Our country has much to gain from these methods. Wage earners would save large sums if, through these treatments, they could continue working. Industry too, which sustains great losses from the incapacitation of part of its labor force, would benefit from workers' improved health. The future, I repeat, lies in education and research.

As for education, this book aspires to that end. Unfortunately, many agencies of the medical profession have refused to budge from their position on steroids, thereby hindering the efforts of those who advocate bee venom. Where is the sociomedical agency that, once medical science in America recognizes the significance of the new method, will dramatically initiate the badly needed, nation-wide program of treatment and research to bring us at least abreast of other countries that are already using these methods?

Education, as a rule, follows on the heels of research. Yet none of the immense sums now being spent for research on arthritis and rheumatism is devoted to research on the honey bee. I will quote a few facts in this regard. In 1959, the United States government appropriated a total of $294.1 million for medical research. Of that sum, $31.2 million (or little more than 10 per cent) was given to cover the study of arthritis and other metabolic diseases. If one penny of that sum was spent on the medications for arthritis and rheumatism which medical science has been advocating for the past 50 years, that one penny was wasted (and almost all of the money is so spent, sad to say).

Gold salts, fever serums, cortisone, hydrocortisone, butazolidin, prednisone, prednisolone, dexamethasone, as well as other hormone and steroid derivatives—not one of them cures arthritis or rheumatism. It is not even claimed that they do so. While they serve as analgesics, so does aspirin, without the drug danger. In fact, plain aspirin has proved superior to the steroids in many studies.

This author has long maintained that research with the honey bee is only in its infancy. No one knows yet how much more benefit to mankind we may secure from the bee. For instance, I have felt for a long time that diseases such as muscular dystrophy might benefit from bee venom treatments.

MEDICAL RESEARCH MONEY

Here is a table showing how much money the National Institutes of Health were allotted for the fiscal year of 1959, the total amount they say they can "effectively" use in 1960 and the amounts voted by the House and Senate:

NAME OF INSTITUTE	1959 BUDGET	COULD USE IN 1960	HOUSE VOTED	SENATE VOTED
	(in millions of dollars)			
Cancer	75.2	84.4	83.3	110.2
Heart	45.6	53.8	52.7	89.5
Mental Health	52.4	61.5	60.4	79.9
Arthritis & Metabolic Disease	31.2	38.7	37.7	51.2
Neurological Disease Blindness	29.4	34.2	33.6	48.9
Allergy & Infectious Disease	24.0	31.1	30.2	41.0
Dental Research	7.4	10.0	9.7	10.1
General Research	28.9	37.5	36.4	49.5
Grand Total	294.1	351.2	344.0	480.3

NOTE: Institutes have about $5 million of 1959 money left as they couldn't spend certain earmarked funds without wasting them. Amounts above represent total for each institute, which includes money for nonresearch purposes too.

American lack of research in the use of bee venom (I have polled many research organizations and found that none of them has ever done any such research) is directly contrasted to the impressive amount of research conducted in Russia and Czechoslovakia. They have done work not only in rheumatism and arthritis but also in a variety of internal diseases which I have long thought would be amenable to bee venom treatment.

In this volume, I have reported on 40 cases which were benefited by treatment with bee venom. A striking fact is that 38 out of the 40 had received steroid treatment in various institutions and from different physicians without any relief, but they *were* benefited by the bee venom injections.

The entire clinical picture of a patient with arthritis or rheumatism is totally different under the treatment with bee venom. There are no relapses after the treatment has been discontinued. No maintenance treatment is necessary. The patient is not subjected to lifelong medical care or treatment.

The general practitioners who read my articles in *General Practice* have responded very enthusiastically. We have not yet been able to catch up with the flow of requests for further information. More research, more treatment of sufferers and more articles are needed.

The makers of the steroids still use the same "ballyhoo" propaganda even though we know that the latest product has the same, and even new, faults that the preceding one had.

We have a serious situation facing us. We must ask ourselves the important question whether the specialists are interested enough to teach the steroid technique to the general practitioner? The next question is whether the general practitioners could learn a technique which the specialists claim is very difficult, consumes a great deal of time and which the specialists themselves have not yet mastered? Finally, with the patient in the middle of this muddle, all he has to look up to is the "noble" Madison Avenue fund-raising slogan of "Let's Stop Arthritis and Rheumatism."

Yes, let's. But how, by whom, when and where do we stop it is still a deep mystery. As yet it isn't a problem of stopping anything, but of starting something. And I am sincerely trying to do just that.

This writer has diligently read the American and foreign literature on bee venom and found it almost uniformly favorable. In one or two instances, the American reports contained some skeptical observations, but these may perhaps have been due to faulty technique used or to some other factors which I point out in the Appendix. Surely, research and clinical work with bee venom ought to be continued and greatly increased.

As we have previously indicated, the research and clinical work comes from such great centers as the Second Medical University Clinic, Munich; the First Medical University Clinic, Vienna; the University Polyclinic, Lausanne; the Lainz Old People's Home for Incurables, Vienna; the Rheumatism Institute, Vienna; the Hospital of the City of Munich in Wessobrunn; the Neurological Clinic, Bucharest; The A. Zimmer Research Institute for Combatting Rheumatism, Berlin; the New York Hospital and the Department of Medicine of Cornell University Medical College, New York; Orthopedic Department, Pembury Hospital, Pembury, Kent, England; London Neurological Clinic, England; Almeric Paget Institute, Islington, England; British Red Cross Clinic for Rheumatism, Peto Place, England; Royal Free Hospital, London; University Eye Clinic, Kiel; Medical Clinic, State Hospital, Nordstadt, Hannover; First Medical Clinic, University of Cracow, Poland; Orthopedic Hospital, Vienna; State Friedrich-Wilhelms-Hospital, Berlin; State University of Gorki, U.S.S.R.; Institute of Medicine, Kharkov, U.S.S.R.; Charles University of Prague, Czechoslovakia; Ambulatorio Medico Mussolini, Bucharest; Second Department of Internal Medicine of the General Polyclinic at Vienna; Anatomical Institute of the Vienna University; Clinic for Rheumatism of the Arbeiter Krankenkasse der Buchkaufmannschaft, Vienna.

We have already delayed too long in further research. Europe has an excuse for little research being done on bee venom for the last 15 years; the war completely disrupted their research programs and facilities. We have few excuses, except possibly unwillingness and apathy.

I hope that by now you are convinced my efforts are in the public interest. You have a duty to help yourselves and others feel the full benefit of bee venom. Together, we can open doors to happiness and health for many of our fellow citizens.

You can help by *demanding bee venom treatments* for arthritis and rheumatism from your physician. Continue your demands until you are satisfied. If he persists in evading or refusing your demands, find another, more progressive physician, of whom there are many, who will give you this treatment which you deserve. Any physician can secure from me all the information needed. He has only to send me a large, stamped, self-addressed envelope. There is no further expense entailed.

Those physicians in the vicinity of New York who wish

to see the treatment and technique actually demonstrated, in addition to the literature I can send them, should come to my office only once for one or two hours in one afternoon and have such a visual demonstration given them, free of charge and without obligations.

Understandably, I cannot answer queries from laymen, as this treatment must be conducted under medical supervision. It's up to you to see that your doctor at least reads the overwhelming preponderance of evidence that rheumatism and arthritis can be cured or dramatically relieved.

BIBLIOGRAPHY

Ackerman, D. and Mauer, H. "About Bee Venom and Its Relation to Histamin." *Pflueger's Arch. ges Physiol,* 247: 623-631, 1944.

Ainlay, G. W. "The Use of Bee Venom in the Treatment of Arthritis and Neuritis." *Nebraska Medical Journal,* 24: 298-303, 1939.

Antonov, J. P. and Boldina, N. A. "Bee Venom Therapy in Some Diseases." *Public Health in Byelorussia,* 12, pp. 44-46, 1956.

Antonov, J. P. and Boldina, N. A. "The *Bee Venom* Treatment of Patients With Neurological Diseases." Transactions of the Byelorussian Institute of Graduate Studies for Practicing Physicians at Minsk, pp. 300-305, 1958.

Artemov, N. M. "The Biological Principles of the Application of Bee Venom in Medicine." Gorki University, U.S.S.R. In process of publication.

Artemov, N. M. "Bee Venom, Its Physiological Properties and Therapeutic Uses." M.L., p. 188, 1941.

Artemov, N. M. "Comparative Study of the Toxic Action of Bee Venom." Scientific reports of the State University in Gorki, 14, pp. 177-204, 1949.

Artemov, N. M. "The Pharmacological Characteristics of Bee Venom." Part 1: Action on the heart. *Uch. Zap. Gork. Gos. Univ.,* 19, 3-16, 1951.

Artemov, N. M. "The Pharmacological Characteristics of Bee Venom." Part II: Comparative study of the action on tonic striated muscles of the venom of bees, snakes, toads and scorpions. *Uch. Zap. Gork. Gos. Univ.,* 19, pp. 17-24, 1951.

Artemov, N. M. and Turilova, V. "Do Animal Poisons Have a Cholinesterase Like Action or an Anti-Cholinesterase Action?" *Uch. Zap. Gork. Gos. Univ.,* 19, pp. 41-51, 1951.

Artemov, N. M. and Shukhalter, T.A. "Effect of Bee Venom on the coagulation of blood."

Artemov, N. M., Kalinina, T. E. and Mikhailova, Ya. V. "Influence of Bee Venom on the Morphological Composition of the Blood of Mammals." *Uch. Zap. Gork. Univ.,* 19, pp. 53-87, 1951.

Artemov, N. M. and Solovieva, O. F. "The Atropin-like Action of Bee Venom." *Bulletin of Exper. Biol. and Med.,* VII, 5, pp. 446-449, 1939.

Arthus, M. "Research Experiments with Bee Venom." *Compt. rend. Soc. de Biolog., Paris,* 182, 1919.

Bacaloglu, C. and Raileanu, C. *Romania Medicala,* #20, 1934.

Balderman, G. "Bee Venom Against Rheumatism." *Medicinische Klinik,* No. 40, 1936.

Bauditsch, H. "Bienenstich." *Prag. Medizin. Wchnschr.,* 31, 1906.

Bayley, de Castro. "The Effects of Bee Venom." *Indian M. Gas.,* Calcutta, 62, 1927.

Beck, Bodog, F. "Bee Venom Therapy." D. Appleton-Century, New York, 1935.

Becker, Siegfried. "Treatment of Rheumatic Diseases With Injectable Bee Venom." *Therapie Der Gegenwart,* Heft 6, 1931.*

Benson, R., and Semenov, H. "Allergy in Its Relation to Bee Stings." *Journal of Allergy,* 1, 1930.

Beylina, P. A. "Acute Poisoning with *Bee Venom* and Its Therapeutic Effect in Rheumatism." *The Soviet Physicians Newspaper,* N7, pp. 546-548, 1934.

Brandt and Ratzeburg. "Die Honigbiene." *Mediz. Zoologie,* 1, 1829.

Brecher, J. "Separate Impression: About Therapeutics with Bee Venom as Remedy of Choice for Trachoma and its Corneal Complications." *Ars Medici: Review for Practical Physicians,* Radauti, Romania, 1934.

Broadman, Joseph. "Local Therapy of Chronic Non-Rheumatoid Arthritis and Rheumatism." The *Journal of the Medical Society of New Jersey,* Vol. 51, p. 320, July, 1954.

Broadman, Joseph. "A New Treatment for Certain Types of Low Back Pain." *American Practitioner and Digest of Treatment,* Vol. 6, No. 8, August, 1955.

* Denotes Kretschy venom, exclusively.

Broadman, Joseph. "Rheumatism and Its Treatment by the General Practitioner." *General Practice,* Vol. 21, No. 5, May, 1958.

Broadman, Joseph. A review of the European literature on the subject of bee venom is cited and the vast amount of clinical and research work in Europe is outlined. *General Practice,* Vol. 21, No. 8, P. 13, August, 1958.

Broadman, Joseph. "Bee Venom for the Treatment of All Types of Rheumatism." A report of 92 cases and case histories is given. Accepted and in process of publication.

Burt, J. B. "Bee Venom Therapy in Chronic Rheumatic Disorders." *British Journal of Physical Medicine,* 12: 171-2, 1937.

Busson, B. *The Bee Venom Therapy.* Book published by Julius Springer, Vienna. 1932.*

Coates, V., and Delicati. "Arthritis and Its Treatment." London, 1931.

Cohen, H., Dubbs, A.W., Pearah, J.B., and Best, C.J. "Bee Venom in the Treatment of Chronic Arthritis." *Pennsylvania Medical Journal,* 45: 957, 1942.

Cohn, S. *Beitraege Zur Kentniss des Bienengiftes.* Inaugural dissertation, Wuerzburg, 1922.

D'Abreu, A. R. "Effects of Bee Venom." *Ind. M. Gaz,* Calcutta, November, 1926.

Devauchelle. "Utilization des Picures d'Abeilles dans le Rheumatisme." *Chasseur Franc.,* October, 1923.

Dimter, Rudolph. "The Treatment of Arthritis with Bee Venom." *Therapie der Gegenwart,* March, 1937.*

Dirr, K. and Graeber, M. "Clinical Judgement of Bee Venom and Its Relationship with Cholesterin Metabolism." *Klin. Wchnschr.*

Elkin, A. C. "Treatment of Osteo-Arthritis." (Scott Method). Medical Press and Circular, No. 5534, May 30, 1945.

Erusalimchik, Kh. I. "Bee Venom Therapy of Sciatic Neuritis and Neuralgia." *Neuropathology and Psychiatry.* Vol. VIII, pp. 36-44, 1939.

Essex, H. B., Markowitz, J., and Mann, F. C. "The Physiological Action of the Venom of the Honey Bee." *American Journal Physiological,* Baltimore, 94, 1930.

Fassenbender, W. "Examinations of the Nature of Bee Venom with the Mercury-drop Cathode." *Biochem. Z.,* 317: 246-255, 1944.

Fehlow, W. "Die Bienengift Behandlung rheumatischer Erkrankungen." *Deutsche Med. Wchnschr,* Berlin u. Leipz., 2, 1934.*

Feldberg, W. "The Action of Bee Venom, Cobra Venom and Lysolecithin on the Adrenal Glands." *Journal of Physiology, 99,* 104, 1940.

Fishkov, E. L. "Therapeutical Uses of the Bee Venom Preparation 'K.F.' " *Clinical Medicine,* XXXII, N8, pp. 20-25, 1954.

Flesch, J. *Technical-Pharmaceutical Journal # 17,* Vienna. *

Flury, F. "About the Chemical Nature of Bee Venom." *Arch. Exper. Pathol. and Pharmacol, 85,* 319, 1920.

Forster, K. A. "About the Sting of the Bee." *Naturwissenschaft,* 11, 1923. *Chemia Medizinische Verwendung Bienengiftes,* 1950.

Freund, E. *Joint Diseases.* Book published by Urban & Schwartzenberg, Vienna, 1929. *

Gaider, F. *Some Experiences in Treatment with Bee Venom.* 2, pp. 43-55, 1955.

Geranke, P., Scheid, G., and Stern, A. "Transcerebrale Bienengiftes Jontophorese bei Arteriellem Hochdruck." *Med. Klinic, 33,* 609, 1937.

Grenfell, M. "The Injectable Bee Venom From the Standpoint of the General Practitioner." *Wiener Med. Wchnschr.,* No. 8, 1932. "Bee Venom and the Public Health." *Arbeiterschutz,* No. 6, June, 1935. *

Grigorescu, D. *Romania Medicala,* No. 6, 1935. *

Guyton, F. E. "Bee Sting Therapy for Arthritis and Neuritis." *Jour. Econ. Entom.,* 40: 469-472, 1947.

Habermann, E., and Moelbert, E., Pharmacological Institute of University of Wuerzburg, Germany. "Morphological Differentiation of Haemolysis with Bee Venom, Snake Venom, Lysolecithin and Digitonin." *Arch. exp. Path. Pharmak.,* 223: 203-216, 1954.

Habermann, E. Pharmacological Institute of University of Wuerzburg, Germany. "Contribution to the Pharmacology of Phospholipase A." *Arch. exp. Path. Pharmak.,* 230: 538-546, 1957.

Hahn, G. and Fernholz, M. E. "About Bee Venom. A Simple Chemical Separation of the Two Venom Components." *Ber. deutsch. Chem. Geselschaft,* 72 (2): 1281-1290, 1939.

Hahn, G., Ostermayer, H., and Ledischke, H. "About Bee Venom." *Berichte Dtsch. Chem. Geselschaft. Mitteilung, 69,* 2, 2764, 1936.

"The Magnesium Content of Bee Venom." *Berichte Dtsch. Chem. Geselschaft, Mitteilung, 70,* 1637, 1937.

Harter, Wolfgang. "Injectable Bee Venom." *Wiener Med. Wchnschr.,* 35-36, 1949.*

Haydak, M. H. "Effect of an Excessive Bee-Stinging." *Minnesota Medicine,* 19: 179-180, 1936.

Heald, C. B. "An Inquiry into the Treatment of Fibrositis." The *Lancet,* London, p. 659, October 13, 1958.

Held, F. *Beitraege zur medizinischer Bedeutung des Bienengiftes.* Inaugural dissertation, Wuerzburg, 1922.

Hellmut, A. "Bee Venom and Immunity." *Z. Immunity,* 105: 241-271, 1946.

Hesse, W. "The Treatment of Rheumatic Diseases with Bee Venom." *Mediz. Monatschr. Heft,* 9, 688, September, 1949.

Istomina, K. V. and Konjevceva, T. V. "The Use of Bee Poison in Polyarthritis" (multiple arthritis). *Sovetskaya Medicina,* 23: 2, 133, 1959.

Jubleau. "Le Traitment du Rheumatisme par Picures d'Abeille." *Chronique Med.,* May, 1925.

Kalinina, L. F. "Comparative Study of the Effects of Animal Poisons on the Morphology of the Blood." *Uch. Zap. Gork. Gos. Univ.,* 1951, 19, pp. 27-39.

Kavetskii, N. E. and Lisunova, M. I. "The Role of Bee Venom Preparations in the Complex Therapy of Patients Suffering from Hypertension and Atherosclerosis." *The Kazan Medical Journal,* 1, pp. 48-53, 1957.

Keiter, A. *Rheumatismus and Bienenschtichbehandlung,* 1914. *Bieneschtichkur, Umschau and Therap. Mon. Bericht.,* 1913.

Kellaway, C. H., Luck, J. M. and Smith, J. H. C. "Bee Venom." *Ann. Rev. Biochem.,* 8: 552-553, 1939.

Kelman, I. M., Sanatoriun Sukhumi, U.S.S.R. "Application of Bee Venom in Sanatorium Conditions." *Pchelovodstvo,* 37 (3); 52-54, 1960.

Kestenbaum, M. *Cernauti Medical,* # 1. 1934.*

Kirchner, E. "Disensitization with Bee Venom in Cases of Allergic Rheumatic Cases." *The Medical World,* # 21, S. 528, 1940.

Koehler, G. "About the Treatment of Chronic Joint Affections with Bee Venom." *Med. Welt,* 43, October, 1932.

Kononenko, L. F. "Bee Venom Preparation 'Melassin' as a Remedy and Disease Preventing Agent." Institute of Medicine, Kharkov, U.S.S.R. In process of publication.

Kononenko, L. F. "Changes in the Hemodynamics of Hypertension and Atherosclerosis Due to Treatment with a Bee Venom Preparation."—Melissisn—Transactions of the Medical Institute of Kharkov, 37, pp. 138-150, 1958.

Kretschy, F. "The Modern Bee Venom Therapy." *Ztschr. f. Wissensch. Baederkunde,* 2, 1928.

Kretschy, Franz. "Bee Venom in Its Historical Development as Therapeutic Agent." *Bienen-Vater,* No. 9, 1928.

Kretschy, Franz. "The Bee Venom." *Bienen-Vater,* No. 7, 1934.

Kroner, J., Lintz, R. M., Tyndall, M., Anderson, L., Nicholls, E. E., "The Treatment of Rheumatoid Arthritis with an Injectable Form of Bee Venom." *Annals of Internal Medicine,* Vol. 16, No. 7, January, 1938.*

Kroner, J. "Rheumatism." Lecture before 3rd International Congress for Rheumatism. October, 1932.*

Lacaillade, C. W., Jr. "The Determination of the Potency of Bee Venom." *Am. J. Physiol.,* Baltimore, 105, August, 1933.

Langer, J. "About the Poison of our Honey Bee." *Arch. Experim. Pathol. and Pharmacol., 38,* 381, 1897 and *4,* 181, 1899. "The Dilution and Destruction of Bee Venom." *Arch. Internat. de Pharmacodyn,* Grand et Par., 6, 1899.

Langer, J. "The Weakening and Destruction of Bee Venom." *Arch. Internat. de Pharmacodyn.* Grand et Par., 6, 1899.

Langer, J. "Bee Venom and the Bee Sting." *Bienen vater.* Jahrg., 33, 10, 1901.

Langer, J. "The Disensitising of the Bee Venom." Address before the German Bee Central Organization, 1898.

Langer, J. "Newer Developments about Bee Stings." Address, Stuttgart, 1930.

Langer, J. "The Fixation of the Bee Venom at the Points of Injection." *Biochem. Ztschr.,* Berlin, 1932.

Laughton-Scott, G. "A New Treatment of Fibrositis." *British Medical Journal,* Vol. 1, p. 302, February 15, 1936.

Laughton-Scott, G. "A New Treatment of Osteoarthritis." *The Practitioner,* Vol. CXL, pp. 307-11, March, 1938.

Laughton-Scott, G. "Local Chemotherapy in Chronic (non-rheumatoid) Rheumatism." *British Medical Journal,* Vol. 2, p. 510, October 23, 1943.

Laughton-Scott, G. "A New Treatment of Osteoarthritis." *The American Journal of Clinical Medicine,* Vol. 54, pp. 85-87, March, 1947.

Laughton-Scott, G. "A Practical Note on Rheumatic Fibrositis." *The Medical Press,* Vol. CCXX, No. 5741, Nov. 10, 1948.

Laughton-Scott, G. "Rheumatic Fibrositis—Some Speculations." *Medical World,* March 7, 1952.

Loebel, R. and Simo, A. "About Ambulatory Treatment of Chronic Joint Diseases, Neuralgias, Myalgias, with Non-Specific Irritation Therapy." *Med. Klin. Berl. u. Wien.,* 10, 1930.*

Lenczner, M. "Treatment of Neuralgia with Bee Venom." *Wiener Medizinische Wochenschrift,* N-14, 1936.*

Lenoch, Frantisek. *Course in Rheumatology,* p. 174, June, 1946.

Lenoch, Fr. *Manual of a Practitioner,* "Injections of Bee Venom, in Rheumatic Diseases," pp. 704-708. "On Immunity to Bee Venom." Vesmir, 29, 107, 1951.

Ludwig, Otto. "The Possibilities in Using Bee Venom in the Treatment of Rheumatic Disorders, Specially Typical and Atypical Gout." *Wiener Klin. Wchnschr.,* 45, 913-16, November 7, 1941.*

Lobachev, S. V., Marenkov, G. M. and Salnikov, V. 1, First Surgical Clinic, Medical Institute, Moscow, U.S.S.R. "Experiments on the Medical Application of Bee Venom." *Pchelovodstvo* 35 (10): 50-52, 1958.

Lordnick, M. "Rheumatism Therapy with Bee Venom." *Aertzliche Practice,* 1954.

Lotter, Georg. "Sensitiveness Against Bee Venom from Typhus and Disensitization with Bee Venom." *Muenchener Medizinischen Wochenschrift,* No. 9, S. 330, 1939.

Lux, Arpad. "Experience with Bee Venom in Arthritis of the Spine." *Mitteilungen Des Verbandes Der Kassenartztlichen Vereine,* Vienna, February, 1937.*

Lyssy, R. "Research Experiments with Bee Venom." *Arch. Intern. de Physiolog.,* 16, 1921.

Maberly, F. H. "Brief Notes on the Treatment of Rheumatism with Bee Stings." *Lancet,* London, July 23, 1910.

Marinescu, B. "Some Data about the Therapeutic Employment of the Bee Venom in Rheumatic Conditions." *Romania Medicala,* 1935.*

Meesmann, A. "About the treatment of Rheumatic Iritis with Bee Venom." *Klinische Monatsblatter fuer Augenheilkunde. Band,* 97. December, 1936.*

Merl, Th. *Zeitschr. f. Untersuchung d. Nahrungs u. Genussmittel,* Berlin, 42, 1921.

Molinery. "Le Traitment du rheumatisme par les piqures d' abeilles." *Chron. Med.,* March, 1925.

Morgenroth, J. and Carpi, W. "Ueber ein Toxolecithid des Bienengiftes." *Berl. Klin. Wchenschr.,* 43, 1906.

Morgenthaler, O. "The Bee Venom Therapy in Rheumatic Diseases." *Schweitz. Bienen Zeit.,* 55: 482, 1932.

Muck, O. "An Overlooked Bee Venom Study." *Wien. Tieraertztlich. Monatshr.,* 1, 1922.

Mueller, E. "The Venom Production of the Honey Bee." *Verhandl. VII Kongress. Entomol.,* pp. 1857-1864, 1938.

Murakami, K. "Influence of Bee's Poison on Blood Picture, Blood Corpuscles, and Cholesterol Content of Blood in Rabbit." *Okayama Igakki Kwai Zasshi,* 40, 1928.

Nasse, H. "News About Bee Venom." *Oestreich. Apoth. Zeitung, Folge* 15, 1953.

Neumann, W. and Stracke, A. "Investigations of Bee Venom and Histamin upon Formaldehyde-Arthritis of the Rat." *Arch. Exper. Pathology and Pharmacology,* 213, 8, 1951.

Neumann, Wilhelm, Ernst Habermann, and Heinke Hansen. "Dif ferentiation of Two Hemolitic Factors in Bee Venom." *Arch. Exper. Pathol. and Pharmacol.,* Vol. 217, S. 130-143, 1953.

Neverova, N. V., Lipetsk Rheumatic Sanatorium for Children. "Use of Bee Venom in Complex Treatment of Chronic Infectious Polyarthritis in Children. *Pchelovodstvo* 35 (6): 45-47, 1958.

Nichols, E. E. "Rheumatoid Arthritis, Treatment with the Sting of the Honey Bee." *New York State Medical Journal,* 38: 1218, 1938.

Nichols, E. H., and Richardson, F. L. "Arthritis Deformans." *Journal of Medical Research,* Boston, 16, 1909.

Nothnagel. "Bee Venom." *Special Pathol. and Therap.,* Vol. 1, 1910.

Novotny, H. "Bee Venom Therapy on Chronically Inflammed Processes." *Muench. Mediz. Wochenschr.,* 29, 1932.*

O'Mahoney, W. W. "Virtues of Bee Venom." *Irish Bee Journal,* 33: 37, 1933.

Ordman, David, South African Institute for Medical Research, Johannesburg. "Bee Sting Sensitivity." *South African Medical Journal,* Vol. 5, pp. 411-413, June, 1951.

Obregia, A. *Romania Medicala,* No. 22, 1935.*

Passow, Pr. "Bee Venom Treatment of Iris Rheumatica." *Klin. Montabl. f. Augenh.,* 79, 1927.

Paul, G. "The Idea of Skin Vaccination and Its Meaning for the Fight Against Chronic Rheumatism." *Wiener Med. Wochenschrift.,* 14, 1927.

Paur, Josef. "Findings with Percutaneous Bee Venom." *Wiener Medicinische Wochenschrift* (#5), 1937.

Perrin, Maurice and Cuenot, Alain. "Rheumatism et Venin d'abeilles." *Congress International du Rheumatisme,* III, Paris, 1932.

Phisalix, M. "Action of Bee Venom on Reptiles and Their Resistance to the Venom." *Ann. Sci. Nat. Zool.,* 10 ser. 18: 67-95, 1935.

Pick, J. "Notes Upon the Morphological Effects of Bee Venom in Vitro and Post-Mortem Experiments." *Wiener Klin. Wochenschr.,* No. 45, 1937.*

Podolsky, E. "The Use of Bees in Medicine." *New York Medical Journal,* November, 1930. *Medicine Marches On,* 1934.

Polak, B. "Bee Venom." *Pharmacology,* p. 144, 1950.

Pollack, H. "About Bee Venom Treatment of Iritis Rheumatica." *Klin. Monatsbl. f. Augenh.,* 81, November, 1928.

Poriadin, V. T., Second Moscow State Medical Institute, U.S.S.R. *Pchelovodstvo,* 35 (8): 49-54, 1958.

Poriadin, V. T. Moscow Medical Institute, U.S.S.R. "Bee Venom Treatment of Diseases of the Arteries of Limbs." *Pchelovodstvo,* 37 (4): 56-57, 1960.

Raileanu, C. *Romania Medicala,* No. 20, 1934.*

Reinert, M. "On the Knowledge of Bee Venom." *Schweitz, Med. Wchenschr.,* 67, 515, 1937.

Reinwand, J. Lecture on Bee Venom given before the Therapy Congress, Karlsruhe, 1952.

Roch, M. "Le Venin d'abeille dans le traitment des Sciatiques." *Rev. Med. de la Suisse Rom. Genève,* February, 1933.

Ross, K. A., Mayer, J. H., Shepherd, M. M. "Osteoarthritis of the Knee. Treatment by Local Injections of Salicylate Compounds." *British Medical Journal,* Vol. 1, pp. 1040-1043, May 3, 1958.

Schaechter, M. *Arch. Med. Chir. de Province,* Nos. 8-9, 1934.*

Schershevskaya, O. J. "Treatment of Rheumatic Iritis with Bee Venom." *Vest. ophtwalm.,* 28, 3, 43-44, 1949.

Schmidt-Lange, W. "The Germicidal Effect of Bee Venom." *Muench. Med. Wchenschr.,* 83, 935, 1941.

Schwabe, R. "A New Method of Application of Bee Venom in Rheumatic Diseases." *Munch. Med. Wchenschr.,* 81, 1934.

Spengler, R., and Pribert, G. "The Combined Bee Venom-Histamin Employment." *Deutsche Medizinische Wochenschrift,* No. 24, S. 962, 1935.

Stadion. "Contribution to Bee Venom Treatment of Myalgia and Sciatica." *Hippokrates; Zeitschrift fuer Practische Heilkunde. Halle a Saale.*

Starkenstein, E. and Weden, H., Pharmacological Institute, German University of Prague. *Medizinische Klinic,* No. 28. July, 1936.

Stefan, Otto. "The Employment of Bee Venom in Cases of Dental Root Therapy." *Deutsche Zahnaertzlihe Wochenschrift,* No. 38, 1937.

Steigerwald, F. and Maurer, M. "Comments on the Treatment of Rheumatism." *Mediz. Wochenschr.,* 8, 581, 1954.

Strasser, A., chairman, medical division of the General Polyclinic, Vienna, Austria, 1928.*

Terc, Philip. "About a Remarkable Connection of Bee Venom with Rheumatism." *Wien. Med. Presse,* 35, 1888.

Terc, Philip. "The Bee Sting as a Remedy Against Rheumatism." *Stierischer Bienenvater,* 1, 1904.

Terc, Philip. "The Action of Bee Stings in Rheumatism and Gout of the Joints," 1910.

Tertsch, R. *Das Bienengift im Dienste der Medizin,* 1912.

Tetsch and Wolff. *Biochem. J.,* 288, 126 (1936); 290, 394 (1937).

Thompson, F. "About Bee Venom." *Lancet,* London, 2, August 19, 1933.

Tigges, W. "Newer Therapy for Neuralgies and Neuritis." *Progress in Therapy,* folio 8, page 250, 1941.

Vigne, P., et Bougala. "Amelioration dans un Cas de Lepre et dans un Cas d'Ulcerede Jambe par les Picures d'Abeilles." *Marseille Med.,* 60, 1923.

Vojtik, V. F. "On the Use of Bee Venom in Internal Diseases." *Clinical Medicine,* 36:9, 131-135, 1958.

Walch, J. "The Treatment of Rheumatic Diseases with Bee Venom Through Intracutaneous Injections." *Revue Medicale de la Suisse,* Part 5, May 25, 1943.

Wasserbrenner, K. "About the Treatment of Rheumatic Diseases with Bee Venom." *Wien. Klin. Wchenschr.,* 35, 1928.*

Weichardt, W. "Studies with Bee Venom." *Deutsche Mediz. Wochenschr.,* No. 37, p. 1405, 1937.

Weidman, M., and Moeller, E. "The Effect of Bee Venom upon the Pituitary-Suprarenal System of the Rat." *Arch. Exper. Pathol. and Pharmacol.,* 220, 465, 1953.

Yoannovitch, G. and Chahovitch, X. "Le Traitment des Lumeurs par le Venin des Abeilles." *Bull. Acad. de Med. Par.,* June, 1932.

Yorish, N. P. "The Pharmacological Properties of Honey and Bee Venom." M., 1952.

Zaitsev, G. P. and Arkhangelskii, A. A. "On the Use of Bee Venom in the Surgical Clinic and the Mechanics of Its Action." *The New Archives of Surgery,* N5, pp. 42-45, 1956.

Zaitsev, G. P. and Poriadin, V. T. "The Use of Bee Venom Therapy in Surgical Diseases." *Apiculture,* 2, pp. 47-50, 1958.

GLOSSARY

ADRENAL CORTEX	Cortical substance of the adrenal gland
AGGLUTINATION	The state of being adherent
AGRANULOCYTOSIS	Destruction of the white cells (granular leucocytes) following an acute febrile disease
ALLERGY	Acquired sensitivities to drugs and biologicals
ANKYLOSIS	Stiffness or fixation of a joint
ARRYTHMIA	Absence of rhythm
ARTHRITIS DEFORMANS	A general term sometimes used to mean any chronic rheumatoid or degenerative arthritis
ATHEROSCLEROSIS	A form of simple arteriosclerosis with deposits within the walls of blood vessels
BILATERAL	Pertaining to, or affecting, both sides of the body
BRACHIAL	Refers to the brachial nerve in the arm
BRACHIAL NEURALGIA	Severe paroxysmal pain along the course of the brachial nerve
CALCIFICATION	Deposit of calcium in the bones and/or joints
CATABOLISM	The series of changes by which living matter or protoplasm breaks down into less complex and more stable substances within a cell or organism
CERVICAL AREA	Around the neck

CLIMACTERIC	A period of life at which the system is believed to undergo marked changes
CORTICOSTEROIDS	A steroid; a form of cortisone
CORTICOTROPIN	A steroid; a form of cortisone
DECALCIFICATION	To free or deprive the bones of calcium
DEXAMETHASONE	A steroid; a form of cortisone
DIABETOGENIC	Diabetes-inducing
DORSAL	Pertaining to the back
DORSIFLEXION	Bending of the foot to stretch the sciatic nerve) located in the lower portion of the back)
ECCHYMATIC SKIN LESIONS	Purple skin blotches
EDEMA	Excessive accumulation of fluid in the tissue spaces
ENDOCARDITIS	Inflammation of the lining of the heart
ENDROCRINOLOGICAL	Relates to glands of internal secretion
ENZYME	A catalytic substance formed by living cells and having a specific action in promoting a chemical change
EPICONDILITIS	Inflammation of the epicondyle of the humerus bone in the arm
EXTENSOR CARPI RADIALIS LONGUS	A muscle in the forearm
FIBROSITIS	An inflammation of muscle tissue
GASTROCNEMIUS	A muscle above and below the knee
GLUTEAL	Pertaining to buttock
HEMORRHAGIC	An escape of blood from the vessels
HIRSUTISM	A condition characterized by the growth of hair in unusual places or in unusual amounts
HYDROCORTISONE	A steroid; a form of cortisone
HYPERCHOLESTERINEMIA	High blood cholesterol
HYPEREMIA	An increased content of blood in a part
HYPERTHYROIDISM	An abnormal condition due to excessive function of the thyroid gland
HYPERTRICHOSIS	Excessive growth of normal hair

HYPERTROPHIC	An increased size of an organ
HYPOTHYROIDISM	A morbid condition due to deficiency of thyroid hormone
IMMUNITY	A condition of a living organism whereby it resists and overcomes infection
INFARCT	A region of destroyed tissue due to complete interference with blood flow
INTRACUTANEOUSLY / INTRADERMALLY	Within the layers of the skin
IRITIS	An inflammation of the iris in the eye
LASÈGUE TEST	A test for sciatica
LESION	An alteration of structure, or of functional capacity, due to injury or disease
LUMBAR REGION	The lower back
LUMBO-SACRAL AREA	The lower back
MENNELL TEST	A test for sacroiliac disease
MILIARY	Characterized by the rapid formation of numerous lesions the size of a millet seed
MOON FACE	Round, edematous face produced by continued use of the steroid hormones such as cortisone
MORPHOLOGIC CHANGES	Cellular change
MYOCARDIAL	Relating to the muscular tissue of the heart
NEUROTOXIC	A toxin capable of destroying nerve tissue
NODULE	A small node
OMARTHRITIS	Inflammation of the shoulder joint
OSTEOARTHRITIS	A chronic arthritis usually involving more than one joint
OSTEOPOROSIS	An enlargement of the spaces of bone; the loss of bony substance
PAPULE	A small, circumscribed, solid elevation of the skin
PATHOLOGY	That branch of biological science which deals with the nature of disease
PATRICK TEST	A test for hip disease

PERIARTHRITIS	Inflammation of tissues about a joint
PERIARTICULAR	Around a joint
PERICARDITIS	An inflammation of the sac enveloping the heart
PERIPHERAL	The external surface
PETERSEN TEST	A test for sacroiliac disease
PHENYLBUTAZONE	A hormone used for treating arthritis and rheumatism
PHYSIOLOGICAL	Pertaining to natural or normal processes as opposed to those that are pathologic
PLAQUE	A patch
POLYARTHRITIS	Inflammation of many joints
POLYNEURITIS	Simultaneous involvement of several nerves, either degenerative or inflammatory
PREDNISOLONE	A steroid; a form of cortisone
PREDNISONE	A steroid; a form of cortisone
PROTEOSE	One of a group of derived proteins intermediate between food proteins and peptones
PYREXIA	Fever
ROENTGENOGRAM	X-ray
SCIATICA	A disease characterized by neuralgic pain along the course of the sciatic (lower back) nerve
SEDIMENTATION	The process of producing the deposition of a sediment
SEPSIS	A general reaction, usually febrile; the result of action of bacteria or their products, or both
SOMATIC	Pertaining to the body
SPONDYLITIS	Inflammation of the spine
SPONDYLITIS DEFORMANS	Ankylosing spondylitis
SUBCUTANEOUSLY	Beneath the skin
SUBOXIDATION	Deficiency of oxygen
SUPRACLAVICULAR FAT PADS	Refers to fat pads above the clavicle around neck ("Buffalo Hump")

SYNDROME	A group of symptoms and signs which, when considered together, characterize a disease or lesion
TACHYCARDIA	Excessive rapidity of the heart action
THROMBOPHLEBITIS	Inflammation of a vein associated with thrombosis
THROMBUS	A clot of blood formed within the heart or blood vessels, usually due to a slowing of the circulation or to alteration of the blood or vessel walls
THYROTOXICOSIS	Hyperthyroidism of any type
TOPICAL	Local
TRAUMATIC	Pertaining to, or caused by, a wound or injury
TRIGEMINAL NEURALGIA	Inflammation of the facial nerves
WHEAL	A primary lesion of the skin which is a circumscribed, edematous, usually transitory elevation

APPENDIX A

Local Therapy of Chronic Nonrheumatoid Arthritis and Rheumatism *

by Joseph Broadman, M.D.

This clinical report describes, with case histories, a method of treating certain types of nonrheumatoid arthritis and rheumatism which has brought promising results in hundreds of patients.

The method was developed by Dr. G. Laughton-Scott, a distinguished London (England) physician, who died in April 1953, after more than 20 years of research in the treatment of rheumatic diseases. Prior to his death, Dr. Scott had drafted plans for introducing his technique to America, and his passing doubtless is one reason why his method is still comparatively unknown in this country.

The Scott method has produced results in the treatment of the following: fibrositis, sciatica, brachial neuritis, intercostal neuralgia, and osteoarthritis.

The therapy consists of weekly injections, for about six weeks, of a 5 per cent solution of camphor and salicylates in oil. As a rule it is possible to discharge patients after approximately six treatments. The dosage varies with the severity. Frequently, less than six treatments suffice; rarely, more than six are needed.

The drugs used are devoid of the dangers inherent in certain drugs and hormones now employed. However, a thorough

* Reprinted from the July, 1954, issue of *The Journal of the Medical Society of New Jersey*, Vol. 51, p. 320.

knowledge of the technic is the key to successful treatment. Mapping of the rheumatic geography must be exact and complete. Patients cannot be entirely relieved if a single lesion is overlooked. Ordinary physical treatment does not demand the same meticulous definition. Idiosyncrasy does not occur with this method, though tolerance may vary. Malaise and pyrexia may follow the initial treatments, but the effects soon pass. Actual pain, if any, can be controlled easily with simple analgesics. With the proper technic and correct doses, the prognosis of the types of rheumatic disease to which this treatment applies become markedly improved.

The actual technique can best be learned while observing its application by someone already experienced with it.

TECHNIQUES

In cases of rheumatic fibrositis the injections are made deep into the tissues, so that the medication spreads over the periosteum, close to the bony origin of the affected muscles. A long enough 19 gauge needle should be used. Each fibrositic lesion must be treated separately. As many lesions are treated at one time as the patient can tolerate. Accurate surface marking for determining the site of injections in relation to the signs and symptoms determines the results.

With rheumatic sciatica the injections are made deep into the gluteal muscles, at the sciatic notch, directly into the periosteum of the notch. Drawing a line between the top of the greater trochanter of the femur and the tuberosity of the ischium, the injections are made at a point between the inner and middle thirds of that line. At the same time, an injection is made to the transverse process of the fourth and fifth lumbar vertebrae of the affected side.

With brachial neuritis, we find the point of severest pain upon pressure on either side of the cervical vertebrae. The injections are made directly into the deep tissues as far as the bony structures underneath, about one half inch from the median line in order to avoid the spinal column.

With intercostal neuralgia, we locate the point of greatest pain and inject into the muscle down to the periosteum of the corresponding rib. Care should be taken not to puncture the pleura.

Osteoarthritis is treated by injections directly into the affected joint. In the knee it is made on either side of the ligamentum patellae, the knee being flexed to as nearly 90 degrees as possible. In the shoulder joint the injections can be made from the front, one half inch outside and one half inch below the coracoid process of the scapula, with the arm rotated outwardly. A similar procedure is followed with other joints.

In all instances, the injection of a local anesthetic should precede each treatment, except in the knee joint, where none is needed. Only when it is necessary to inject directly into the thick parts of the ilium, the top of the tibia, the top of the femur or into the occiput, is a general anesthetic needed. Similarly, whenever mass injections are given, general anesthesia should be employed. A finer needle is used when injecting smaller joints.

A definitive evaluation of the Scott method had been incorporated in the report of a special committee of the London Medical Society in 1951. This report was the outgrowth of a clinical study made by four eminent specialists appointed by the Society in 1949 to make a thorough inquiry into Dr. Scott's method. Two years were required to complete the study. During this period the four physicians treated about 200 cases of fibrositis, using the method described by Dr. Scott. At the completion of the clinical study, the committee submitted a report to the Society stating that 78.5 per cent of the cases treated by them were either "free of symptoms" or "plus improved." The entire group of patients was followed up, some as long as 15 months and at the time the report was rendered, the committee found that there had been no change in the condition of any of the patients since discharge. The committee's report was published in the *Lancet* which stated in part:

The average duration of symptoms was 3.1 years: the average number of injections per case was 5.9 and the average follow-up time 8.9 months (minimum 6 and maximum 15). The long interval between the end of treatment and the follow-up, seems to us to enhance the significance of the improvement recorded.

The injections were given once a week, unless the patient had a strong reaction accompanied by malaise. This malaise appeared in so many cases during treatment, and was so often followed by freedom from symptoms or "plus improvement" that we came to look on its appearance as a favorable sign. We noted also that when the reactions cleared up the majority of patients volunteered the statement that their general health had improved. When similar injections were made in 14 healthy volunteers, none had either reactions or malaise.

Our impression—supported by our figures as far as they go—is that patients treated by this method are relieved sooner, attend hospital less often, and have less disability than patients treated by other methods. In uncomplicated cases of fibrositis this method seems to relieve symptoms for longer periods than others familiar to us.

COMMENTS

Based on the writer's clinical experience, it is sugegsted that local chemotherapy of chronic arthritis and rheumatism with camphor and salicylates in oil is an effective treatment and an advance over existing methods. Emphasis is placed on the need for extreme accuracy in locating the rheumatic lesion before it is attacked. Not all osteoarthritic joints respond to this treatment in the same degree.

The Scott technique shortens disability time, the patient rarely requiring more than six treatments, all of which can be administered by the physician in his office. Only such patients who have too many lesions for office treatment, or who desire quicker results through massive treatments, need hospitalization or nursing home care.

Reactions consisted of malaise and pyrexia, in some cases, which passed in 24 to 48 hours. Pain, if any, can easily be controlled by simple measures. No infections or complications were noted. The usual aseptic precautions were followed.

APPENDIX B

Rheumatism and Its Treatment by the General Practitioner *

by Joseph Broadman, M.D.

The classification of rheumatic diseases used in this country has not yet been accepted everywhere, because frequent overlaps create much confusion. Those rheumatic diseases whose causative agent is unknown, overlap even more often. These uncertainties make accurate diagnosis by the general practitioner very difficult.

Rheumatism and arthritis can be dealt with effectively by the general practitioner in a much simpler manner than heretofore attempted. According to this plan, the nomenclature can be narrowed down to just two groups of rheumatic diseases, namely, (a) those for which the causative agent is known and (b) those whose cause is unknown. Since modern types of treatment are enumerated here for each of the two groups, such a division would reduce the subject to simplicity itself. It will make it possible for each general practitioner to help many of his patients who have so far resisted all other kinds of treatment, and this applies mainly to the group of rheumatic diseases for which the causative factor is still unknown.

It has been estimated that there are at least 11,000,000 rheumatics in the United States.

A two group division would consist of:

1. Rheumatic and arthritic diseases due to known causative agents as tubercular arthritis and spondylitis; gonococcal

* Reprinted from *General Practice,* May, 1958, Vol. 21, No. 5.

arthritis; luetic and gummatous arthritis; Charcot's joint; brucellosis; meningococcus arthritis; rheumatic fever; and some others of less importance.

The above types of rheumatic diseases can be diagnosed with comparative ease by the mode of onset, the history, manner of exposure, its location, age of patient, progress of the condition and a thorough physical examination. Laboratory tests are frequently necessary. Such patients usually show fever and an increased number of leucocytes. The sedimentation rate is frequently elevated. Blood culture, synovial fluid or smear examinations often reveal the causative microorganism. Inoculations of guinea pigs, if necessary, can be resorted to. Examination of the lymph nodes may help. In some types of cases, in their later stages, X-ray may be of service, as for example in tuberculosis.

Once the offending microorganism is found and a diagnosis made, the physician surely will know that for the treatment of tubercular conditions, streptomycin comes into play, unless surgery is indicated; for gonococcal conditions, penicillin seems best, with streptomycin and aureomycin, in penicillin-resistant patients next; for meningococcus infections, sulfonamide compounds orally and penicillin intramuscularly are used; for lues and Charcot's joint, penicillin is useful and, if necessary, arsenic and bismuth come into play; for brucellosis, streyptomycin, aureomycin and sulfonamide compounds are useful; for rheumatic fever, adequately large doses of acetyl-salicylic acid and sodium salicylate are considered specifics. Penicillin and sulfonamide drugs are also useful.

Other means at our disposal, such as bed rest, proper diet, active and passive motion, massage and proper support should be employed as soon as the temperature returns to normal and the local symptoms have subsided. This is of even greater importance in the later stages to prevent ankylosis and deformity as well as to restore function. Most other infectious processes are sensitive to one or another of the antibiotics or sulfonamides.

We now come to the more important group of rheumatic

diseases whose causation is still unknown. They are the group two in our scheme of things and they include:

2. Rheumatoid arthritis; rheumatoid spondylitis; degenerative or osteoarthritis; gout; nonarticular rheumatic diseases, such as fibrositis and other less important conditions.

Whatever may be the cause of the diseases in group two, that cause seems to be operating in various strains and severities. One of these strains causes rheumatoid arthritis, another causes rheumatoid spondylitis or osteoarthritis, while still another results in gout. The weakest of the strains brings about the nonarticular rheumatic conditions. *Basically,* they all appear to belong to the same family of disease-causing agents, or so many of them would not overlap as they do.

Furthermore, because they are of the same family of diseases, caused by the same family of agents, one type of treatment favorably affects them all.

Bee venom, when properly administered under proper conditions, will benefit many cases of the diseases in this group two. This one remedy can be used freely, in all those conditions, without going into the fine distinguishing, diagnostic points heretofore looked for as a prerequisite to treatment. Severe and chronic cases require the use of the strongest concentrations and the longest time and patience, while average or mild cases need less time and patience, and the use of milder concentrations. Recent cases naturally bring the best results. This is actually how simplified the treatment can be made, if before beginning the treatment less than five minutes are taken to test for allergy.

ORIGIN OF CONCEPT

It has been known for many centuries that keepers of beehives were free from arthritis and rheumatism, and in the public mind this has been ascribed to the repeated stings of those keepers by the honey bee. Some physicians of ancient and more recent times also accepted the fact that the stings of bees had a favorable effect in preventing arthritis and rheumatism and in curing it when it had already developed. To treat humans with live bee stings, however, is rather crude. Today, the *bee venom* has been isolated, purified and even standardized. It can now be administered like any other modern, scientific medication. Many doctors and patients, running into the tens of thousands, have already been treated with this method, without any side effects, complications or fatalities.

While a great many people, including physicians, have read about *bee venom* at one time or another, little has been published of the details. Those who have had experience with *bee venom* praise it most highly.

In the November and December, 1956, issues of *Annals of Internal Medicine,* published by the American College of Physicians, the Editorial Committee of the American Rheumatism Association published its Eleventh Rheumatism Review of American and English Literature of the three most recent years. That report filled 265 pages and, therefore, had to be split into two issues of the journal.

Presenting a detailed picture of the effects from the use of various hormones and steroids, the report is full of much valuable information. A few quotations from the report are cited here, as follows:

"Untoward Effects. Much attention was devoted to the undesirable effects which develop during treatment with corticotropin or corticosteroids. The frequency of such undesirable effects varied in different series from 23% to 65%; and they were seen to some extent in 83% of 36 essentially normal young men treated with substantial amounts of ACTH or cortisone for 31 consecutive days. Determining factors appeared to be dosage, duration of treatment, individual susceptibility, and nature of the disease treated.

"The potential hazards of long-term therapy with ACTH and cortisone were emphasized by a study of the natural history of Cushing's syndrone. The clinical course of 212 patients with spontaneous hyperadrenalism was characterized by a high incidence of mental abnormalities, poor wound healing or unusual intercurrent infections. In 114 autopsied cases, the major causes of death were infection, cardiovascular disease, and neoplastic disease. An extremely high incidence of arteriosclerosis and osteoporosis was noted."

They go on to report "in several series of patients the frequency of distinctly aberrant psychologic reactions was 5.5% of 128 patients, 6.3% of 63 patients, and 15% of 66 and of 80 patients, respectively. Most of the psychoses were mild, transient and self limited when the hormones were withdrawn, but some required shock therapy."

Numerous reports of activities of duodenal ulcers during cortisone or corticotropin therapy have been reported. In some cases there were no previous ulcer histories. The ulceration was often first manifested as a complication, such as perforation or hemorrhage. "Of 18 cases reviewed from the literature, 12 manifested perforation, hemorrhage, or both; there were five deaths from complications of peptic ulcer. Gastrointestinal bleeding also occurred in the absence of lesions demonstrable by X-ray."

The incidence of toxic reactions to phenylbutazone was high. In a series of 800 patients—40% developed some evidence of toxicity; this was severe enough to require discontinuation of the drug in 15% of the 800. Review of the literature prior to June, 1953, yielded an average of 22% of 1,526 patients who experienced toxic reactions. Gastrointestinal symptoms, most commonly nausea, diarrhea or constipation, occurred in 15% or more of patients. Agranulocytosis was held responsible for seven deaths and occurred in at least 20 additional patients who recovered following discontinuation of the drug and the use of antibotics.

Where phenybutazone is used, careful selection of patients and close attention to signs of toxicity should be demanded.

Much more could be written regarding the complications, side effects and even deaths with some of the treatments pursued. A comparison of the records of the results from the use of hormones and steroids and *bee venom* indicates clearly the course that ought to be pursued. I cannot avoid reaching the conclusion that *bee venom* merits the careful consideration of the general practitioner.

It is not claimed that this form of treatment will cure each patient. What has been shown is that large numbers of patients can get substantial relief. Many early cases will obtain permanent relief, while others will get only partial results, depending upon the duration, chronocity and the amount of pathology. A very few will not benefit at all.

Bee venom has as its additional advantage a simplicity of use that lends itself to the practice of all general practitioners wherever they may be. Under the method of treatment here recommended, the smallest community in the country could secure these advantages for its afflicted. The general practitioner could in a short time become as well trained and equipped as the best of us.

* * *

The reaction from general practitioners who read the article in *General Practice* was encouraging. The normal office personnel of the journal was unable to cope with the flood of ensuing mail. To satisfy the demand for further information, the editor asked me for a follow-up article. Following publication of the second article, mail continued to flood my office, as well as the publisher's office. As printed in the magazine, here is a sampling of such correspondence.

GENTLEMEN:

Today I received my "first" issue of *General Practice.* I immediately became interested in it and read it almost in its entirety.

In my opinion, it is one of the finest and best journals of its kind.

Thank you very much for sending it to me. I will be looking forward for the future issues to come.

While reading this General Practice journal I came across the article entitled, "Rheumatism and Its Treatment By the General Practitioner." It was very informative and educational.

This article, written by Joseph Broadman, M.D. (in the May issue), states that *"Bee Venom"* when properly administered under proper conditions will benefit many sufferers of "Rheumatoid Arthritis."

I would greatly appreciate it if you would let me know where this "Bee Venom" is available—what pharmaceutical houses stock it and under what trade name, if any. In addition I would appreciate any and all information in regards to its administration, dosage, etc.

Further, I would appreciate finding out what the author means by "proper administration" and "proper conditions."

If you cannot furnish this information, I would be grateful if you would let me know where I can obtain this information.

Thank you very much. I will be patiently awaiting your reply.

Yours truly,

Thank you for your very fine letter. We appreciate your remarks in regard to General Practice.

Dr. Broadman's paper has certainly brought us a carload of mail and so we are taking the liberty of answering you in print so that everyone who is interested in learning more about Dr. Broadman's treatment will have his address also.

Write to:

Joseph Broadman, M.D.,
55 Central Park West
New York 23, New York.

Thank you again for your friendship.

The Editors

DEAR EDITORS:

I am very pleased to know that your publication of my article on bee venom for the treatment of rheumatism, including rheumatoid arthritis, has brought you an avalanche of inquiries for further information. I, too, have been flooded with such inquiries.

When your readers begin to see the results and when their suffering patients commence to feel the effects of those results, they will all bless you for the service you have rendered to them.

In response to the wide demand for further information on how to apply this therapy, I am preparing the following:

1. I am gathering the necessary literature which will present to the physician the theoretical portion of bee venom therapy, and,
2. In addition, I am ready to give two free, consecutive afternoon

lectures from 2 to 5 o'clock to any physician who comes to my office, which will be devoted to the technical part of the subject. Between the literature and the demonstrations the physician will become competent to treat his own patients. The lectures will be given weekly, either on Monday and Tuesday, or on Thursday and Friday.

I feel that even though the technique is easy to learn, any physician should be willing to spend two afternoons at my office, which will be ample to make him able.

Any physician interested in this free course will please write to me, suggesting which days and weeks will suit him best to come here, and I will accommodate him.

Sincerely yours,
Joseph Broadman, M.D.

GENTLEMEN:

I was very much interested in your August, 1958, issue of "General Practice" in which there appeared an article written by Dr. Joseph Broadman on the treatment of all types of rheumatism by bee venom.

I have tried for the past year to purchase bee venom, but with no success. Will you please send me information as to where or how I can obtain bee venom? Thank you.

Yours truly,

DEAR SIR:

We were pleased to see the article reviewing Bee Venom for the treatment of rheumatism, in the August issue of your magazine, Volume 21, No. 8.

We have been unable to secure Bee Venom for about a year. Drughouses here tell us it is no longer manufactured.

If you have any additional information as to the availability of this medicine, we will appreciate hearing it.

Sincerely yours,

Interest in Dr. Broadman's articles concerning the use of bee venom continues to bring us inquiries from all parts of the nation. And Dr. Broadman is still the best source of further information; he may be addressed (etc.).

APPENDIX C

A Review of the Foreign Literature on Bee Venom for the Treatment of All Types of Rheumatism *

by JOSEPH BROADMAN, M.D.

The basic consideration of the present article is to call attention to the vast amount of research and clinical work done on *bee venom* in various European university centers and reported in the leading medical journals of the respective countries. Comparatively little has been done or published in this country.

The conclusions are clear and inescapable. The major part of the patients responded rather favorably, while only a small fraction experienced lesser relief, and a negligible number of patients derived no benefit at all. Severe joint changes are irreversible; hence treatment should begin before such changes develop.

Considering the methods devised by Dr. Scott and those described here, the physican would have two distinct methods of treatment at his disposal, applicable to the various types of rheumatic diseases. Incidentally, both these methods can be administered conveniently by any physician in his office.

RESEARCH FINDINGS

Dirr and Graeber, in their work at the Second Medical Clinic, University of Munich, have found that the cholesterol content of the blood was greatly increased, following the em-

* Reprinted from *General Practice,* August, 1958, Vol. 21, No. 8.

ployment of *bee venom* in rheumatic cases. Increase of cholesterol was observed neither in healthy persons nor in patients with other diseases than rheumatism and its concommitant complications. It appears, therefore, that this development occurs only in rheumatic cases. The authors suspect strongly the presence of toxic matter in the tissues of rheumatic patients, presumably mobilized by the catalytic action of the *bee venom* used, but rendered harmless by the cholesterol itself.

Feldberg, London, when publishing in 1940 his findings on the subject, discloses the fact that a flow of adrenalin is invariably discharged, following a large dose of *bee venom*.

Weidman and Moeller, Copenhagen, reported in 1953 that the adrenal glands lost much of their ascorbic acid content, following the injection of *bee venom* in healthy animals, a reaction which does not occur in animals stripped of their pituitary gland.

Since like effects have been observed also as following the use of cortisone and ACTH, it appears that the observations made by Dirr and Graeber, Feldberg and Weidman and Moeller indicate the effects of *bee venom* to be similar to cortisone-ACTH reactions. Their conclusions point to the fact that *bee venom* is actually the most modern therapy available.

Although the manner in which the patient reacts to treatment with *bee venom* is still under discussion, general agreement has been reached, however, that it is an agent completely different from any other currently used, and that it has a favorable effect on the entire organism.

Langer, head of the children's clinic at Graz, Austria, reported as far back as 1897-99 on the chemistry of *bee venom*.

Flury, head of the Pharmacological Institute of the University of Wuerzburg, reported in 1920 of his own work on the chemistry of *bee venom*.

Reinert reported in 1937 on the chemistry and physical aspects of *bee venom*.

Hahn, Ostermayer and Ledischke reported in 1936 on the

chemistry of *bee venom* and what we know about the magnesium content of it.

Geranke, Scheid and Stern reported in 1937 on the *Transcerebrale Bienengift-Jontophorese bei arteriellem Hochdruck.*

Schmidt-Lange reported in 1941 on the germicidal effect of *bee venom.*

Neumann and Stracke published in 1951 conclusive evidence of the antiarthritic effect of *bee venom* when same was injected in rats with formaldehyde-induced arthritis.

CLINICAL OBSERVATIONS AND TREATMENT

As will be seen in what follows, the reports of cases I presented in my last article, are not unique. Many other clinical workers were equally successful in their results:

Terc, the father of modern *bee venom* treatment, reported his first 175 cases in 1888. He is the man who used 39,000 live bee stings on his first 175 patients, something present-day physicians do not need to resort to.

Beck, of New York, for many years concentrated on the treatment of all types of rheumatic diseases with *bee venom,* with very satisfactory results. Like Terc, he used the stings of the live honey bee for the purpose. He strove to arouse the profession to the merits of *bee venom.* He sought to bring to their attention the advantages of its use, for those resistant to other types of therapy. Though his efforts met with little success, he did not become disheartened. He made a record of his work and results in a very fine book published in 1935.

The clinicians named in this review used *bee venom* in one of two forms: Terc and Beck used the stings of the live honey bee in their work. However, this was before the advent of the present injectable *bee venom.* All others used the latter, immediately upon its becoming available.

Siegfried Becker at the First Medical University Clinic, Vienna, inaugurated his treatments with *bee venom* with 120 cases of varied types of rheumatic diseases, with satisfactory results. His report was published in 1931. In this report, he dwells in great detail on the technique, mode of treatment, local and general reactions, the relationship of alcohol to the treatment with *bee venom* and many other pertinent facts.

Perrin and Cuenot, France, lectured on the subject before the International Congress on Rheumatism, Paris, 1932. They enumerated a number of prominent French clinicians who employ *bee venom* with satisfactory results.

Marinescu, of the Neurological Clinic, Bucharest, speaks of his good results with *bee venom* in his report of 1935.

Dimter, of the Lainz Old Peoples' Home for Incurables, Vienna, tells a most interesting story in his report of 1937. He speaks of his early skepticism and his agreeable surprises with *bee venom*. His patients were of the worst type, ages between 60 and 80. His results, he states, were beyond expectations.

Kroner, Lintz, Tyndall, Anderson and Nichols served on a team which made a special study of 100 cases of rheumatoid arthritis for the New York Hospital in conjunction with the Cornell University Medical College. This report was published in 1938. Of the 100 cases, 75 improved. The results were so surprising that the team stated, "It would seem, therefore, that *bee venom* is worthy of further consideration."

Ludwig, of the A. Zimmer Research Institute for Combatting Rheumatism, Berlin, in an address made during the third "Viennese Medical Week," in 1941, states that in his polyclinic for rheumatism, the largest in Germany, he has used *bee venom* for the past 14 years on cases of rheumatism and gout in increasing numbers of patients. He gives that fact as the best indication of what he thinks of *bee venom*.

Harter, of the Rheumatism Institute, Vienna, reports on a group of nonarticular cases, such as sciatica, brachial neuritis, migraine, trigeminal neuralgia and intercostal neuralgia. His report was published in 1949. This clinician even gives the number of treatments needed in each case for the best results, which he checked six months after stopping the treatments.

J. Walch, at the Polyclinic of the University of Lausanne,

gives an interesting report of his first 100 cases of many types of arthritic diseases, which was published in 1943. The results of treatment with *bee venom* were very satisfactory.

Reinwand lectured on the subject before the Therapy Congress of 1952 at Karlsruhe and recited the many advantages of *bee venom.*

Steigerwald and Maurer, of the Hospital of the City of Munich in Wessobrunn, Germany, relate their own experiences with the first 100 cases of all types of rheumatism, published in 1954. They also report very satisfactory results.

Much additional clinical work in Europe can be cited. This author, however, feels that the results enumerated and referred to in this paper are sufficient to prove his point.

APPENDIX D

Technique of Bee Venom Treatment

The needles are 27 gauge and one eighth inch long, with very short bevels, obtainable from Becton, Dickinson Company, Rutherford, N. J. The Luer syringe, one to two cc. size, is used. Both the needle and the syringe are held parallel to the skin while injecting.

All bee venom injections are given *intradermally*. The skin should be stretched and the needle inserted quickly. First, cleanse the skin with surgically pure benzine or with a plain soap solution. *Do not use alcohol in connection with any bee venom treatments, either to sterilize or clean instruments,* nor should the patient partake of even one drop of alcohol during the treatments, including patent medicines, for alcohol neutralizes the bee venom and makes the treatments useless. Use sterilization by boiling or autoclaving.

With the patient lying down, begin with one single intradermal injection of one tenth cc. of the weakest bee venom concentration on the upper back, as a test for allergy to the venom, and observe the patient for 15 to 20 minutes. If no serious systemic reaction develops in that time, it means that no allergy is present against bee venom and any symptoms which may develop, local or systemic, will not be of a serious nature.

The injections are administered daily in nonarthritic cases, and every other day in the arthritic types, for we employ the weaker concentrations mostly in the nonarticular (nonjoint) and the stronger concentrations in the articular (joint) types. In the nonarthritic cases, proceed with the treatment, using the weakest concentration, and increase the wheals at each visit by one or two until you reach 20 wheals. By this time the patient usually is fully relieved. Only in stubborn cases does it become necessary to use the next higher concentration; begin with one wheal of this higher concentration and gradually increase the number at each visit until the patient is completely relieved. The last dose which produced the relief should be repeated two or three times, in order to fortify the result obtained. The wheals are usually placed about one inch apart.

In articular types of cases, give about ten more injections (wheals) of the weakest concentration and change over to the next stronger concentration. Gradually increase the number of wheals to 20, when you again go to the next higher concentration and proceed with the gradual increase as before. Recent cases are usually better when medium concentration is reached. In old and stubborn cases, it frequently becomes necessary to go to even higher concentrations until the patient is relieved.

If during treatment, a severe local reaction of increased pain should develop, the size of the last dose should be either maintained or increased, but the treatment should not be relaxed or discontinued. Such reactions are favorable signs, to be anticipated, because they usually are indications that the patient is responding well and will improve more rapidly when the reaction is over—in two or three days.

As the venom enters the skin, a wheal is formed in a matter of seconds, followed by a characteristic reddish ring around it. At first the wheals are round, but they soon begin to change their shapes and become irregular and serrated. This process of change keeps progressing until they gradually fuse with each other to form one huge wheal, called a plaque. When this plaque is formed, give two or three more treatments, consider the patient fully immunized and that particular course of injections ended.

Immunity, however, is never permanent. It wears off. Hence, you should always, no matter how slowly or quickly the patient progressed, follow up the treatment with another course of injections four to six weeks after the first. In this case, however, do not watch the changes in the wheals for their fusion tendencies; the patient is already saturated.

It is of utmost importance to carefully observe and make a record of the characteristics of the wheals in the first course of injections, because they are the vital mirror of the progress made. Note the speed of their development, duration of reaction and their vanishing; and mark those changes for their diagnostic and prognostic value.

Cases of nonarthritic nature rarely need more than one course of injections to bring about complete relief, and they frequently require less. With arthritic cases, it depends upon how recent or chronic the case happens to be. Acute rheumatic fever, with or without endocarditis, responds promptly. Begin with one wheal of the weak concentration, increasing very slowly every other day. As long as the fever lasts, give antipyretics on the off days, but stop them as soon as the temperature approaches normal.

The amount of bee venom used for each wheal is never more than one tenth cc. of the venom. The locations best suited for the injections are the interscapular, lumbar and sacral regions on both sides of the spinal column. With knee, elbow or wrist cases, or any other similar joints, if the pains are very severe, inject into the skin directly over the joints, *but always on the extensor side of the joint,* or marked swellings will result from interference with the lymphatic circulation. Arteries and veins must be avoided. Inject on alternate sides of the spinal column on alternate visits.

APPENDIX E

Russian Correspondence and Papers

Moscow, March 18, 1960

DEAR DOCTOR JOSEPH BROADMAN:

May I express my warm thanks for your nice letter, from February 8, 1960, which I have read with great interest. Excuse me please for writing in Russian, but my interpreter is away on an official mission. I am taking the liberty to give a brief answer to all the questions that interest you.

It would be purposeless in my opinion to translate my works, because they are mostly written in a popular style, and their number exceeds a hundred. My book will appear in French, in the near future, and I shall send it to you as a present. I shall be very glad, if you will like it, and if it will be of any use to you in your noble activity.

Concerning tests with your bee venom tablets, I shall be glad to help with tests and clinical observations. It will be especially interesting, because I have introduced the sublingual method of application of queen's jelly, which has met with the approval of my colleagues in France, China, Roumania, Czechoslovakia, etc. I think, that sublingual application of bee venom will also be found useful. But according to data available to me, the cholesterol level in the blood is depressed by bee venom, while you maintain, on the contrary, that a rise in the cholesterol blood level is a criterion of the bee venom action. You may rest assured, that as soon as I shall receive your tablets I will endeavor to test them, with the help of an objective colleague, in one of the clinical institutions, having the greatest authority. In the spring I will begin to receive fresh apitoxin, and it will be a pleasure to send it to you, in the hope that you will find it possible to communicate your critical observations.

I am happy to know, that you agree with me, that natural bee venom has the most effective therapeutic action. As far as the dosage is concerned, we consider as a unit the whole amount of bee venom contained in the venom bag of one bee and introduced intradermally. A course of treatment consists of 200 bee units. The forceps I propose (see description in N-12 of *Pchelovodstvo,* 1960) makes it possible to introduce in the skin one unit in one second. I consider as criteria of the therapeutic effect subjective symptoms: general well-being, working capacity, etc.; and objective signs: disappearance of the swelling of the joints, auscultation of the heart, electrocardiogram, decreased sedimentation rate and cholesterol in the blood, rise in the permeability of the vessels and lowered blood pressure.

I hope to publish in the near future our method of obtaining bee venom without harm to the bee, and I will send you this paper as soon as it comes out. I work at present on the simplification of this method and I will be happy if it will be widely used for the benefit of the people. . . .

I am very glad that you liked the medal of our section of medical apiculture. Thank you very much for your flattering opinion of my article in *Pchelovodstvo,* which you called "very interesting."

May I express my sincere thanks for your kind cooperation, and my hope, that I shall soon receive your answer.

Respectfully yours,

N. YORISH

(Doctor Yorish is an ardent research worker for the government of Russia in the vast field of Bee Venom therapy; a prolific writer on the general subject of medical apiculture, having written several books, in as many languages, on this subject. A dedicated humanitarian, he is interested not only in helping the people of Russia but of the entire world, and he has already been instrumental in the development of techniques for the employment of Bee Venom in a large variety of diseases other than arthritis and rheumatism, with very considerable results. Aside from all that, he is also the president of the Section of Amateur Medical Apiarists of Russia.)

Moscow, April 18, 1960

DEAR DOCTOR JOSEPH BROADMAN:

May I warmly thank you for your kind and extremely interesting letter with detailed instructions on the use of apitoxin in tablets of your invention. I received also your parcel containing 25 glass containers with apitoxin tablets. Everything was made so beautifully and with such loving care that I was delighted when I opened the package. The very idea to spare the patients painful injections and unpleasant applications of apitoxin, and to give the sufferers the means to use these tablets under any conditions, deserves the gratitude of mankind. I always dreamed of medicines of this kind, which would combine high therapeutic effect with the absence of unpleasant sensations. It is especially important for children.

I am very glad that you approve my plans for laboratory experiments and clinical observations. In case you could find it possible to give your permission, it would be desirable to send some of these apitoxin tablets to my colleagues in Bulgaria, Czechoslovakia and China, so that they in their turn could make the appropriate experiments and clinical observations. Naturally, I shall send them your instructions and point out that *you are the author of this new and interesting therapeutic method.*

As far as the influence of apitoxin on the decrease of cholesterol in the blood is concerned, my opinion is based on our observations. There are, however, scientific papers, for instance Forster and others, where a rise of blood cholesterol is described. I think that just at the present time an exact and final solution of the problem will be achieved and the scientific truth will be victorious.

If it is not too much trouble, may I ask you to answer the following questions:

1. What method do you use to obtain apitoxin?
2. What do the tablets contain besides apitoxin?
3. What kind of dyes are used to color the tablets—vegetable or mineral?

I will be, probably, asked these questions by the Scientific Council of the Ministry of Health, before the permission for clinical experiments is granted. In case these data are secret, may I ask you to answer at least the third question. Sometime later I shall send you a small parcel with those apitoxin preparations which I have used (crystalline Czech Virapine and German Apisartron).

I wish you good health and new creative achievements in your noble activity.

Sincerely yours,
N. YORISH

Krasnokursantsky 7 app. 13
Yorish Naum Petrovich

Professor, Doctor Joseph Broadman
New York

DEAR COLLEAGUE:

I read with the greatest pleasure your kind letter, in which you mention that your book will come out soon. I am very happy for your sake. The publication of a scientific book, or a book of popular science is a great achievement for an author, who wants his method known to physicians and patients. I hope that you will grant me this honour and send me a signed copy of your book. A few weeks ago I sent you my new album "Bees and Health," which you have probably received by now, and will be now able to study and criticize. In the next edition I intend to give many more photographs and drawings illustrating the methods of obtaining apitoxin, so that every physician and/or patient could get bee venom from an apiary or a therapeutic institution the whole year round.

I thank you once more for your New Year's wishes and wish you in return the best of health and great creative successes. I shall let you have all the news about the progress of our exhibition. We have not yet started our experiments with your tablets, but I shall come to an agreement with the Institute of Rheumatology in the near future. I am somewhat confused by the fact that in your first letter you recommended to hold the tablet between cheek and gum for about 10m., then, in your second letter, to hold it about 1 hour, and that you suggest in your last letter to dilute it in lemon juice (at least in some cases).

I want to try your tablets on myself, and to find out the time needed for dissolution and sublingual absorption. It would be interesting to learn the results of your experiments in Czechoslovakia and other countries and in the USA.

As far as the apparatus for making tablets is concerned, the Moscow specialists do not recommend to occupy oneself with it.

Please accept, dear colleague, the expression of my deep regards.

Sincerely yours,
N. YORISH

Moscow, February 18, 1961

To Professor Dr. Joseph Broadman
New York

DEAR COLLEAGUE:

Thank you very much for your kind letter of March 8, 1961, and for the copy of Prof. Lenoch's letter from Prague. I am very happy to hear about your vigorous activities and the impressive results achieved with the sublingual preparation of bee venom which you have introduced. My album "Bees and Health" is sold out and we have started work on a new edition. In this revised edition all sections will be enlarged, especially the one that interests you. I have in mind the chapter "Methods of Obtaining Bee Venom Without Harm to the Bee." At the same time I am preparing for publication a little book "Apitoxinotherapy," in which all the best known methods of apitoxinotherapy will be discussed. I already mentioned in my letters, that contrary to foreign methods in which the toxic protein is eliminated from all bee venom preparations, I have always stressed in my scientific work as well as in practice that the *basic and chief* therapeutic effect is due to toxin protein. The ultimate object of all my endeavors has always been to make all my achievements immediately available to the masses. Pictures representing collection of bee venom, show quite clearly that bees crawling on a window pane, are picked up with tweezers and held over a cover glass so that the bee's belly touches the glass. The bee stings immediately, leaving a drop of venom on the glass, but its sting is left intact, and consequently the bee stays alive. During a 6-hour day one worker on the apiary is able to collect a couple of thousand drops of native bee venom. This method is acceptable to all concerned—apiarists, scientists and, especially, patients. I am striving to improve this method but for the present I am satisfied with the results, because I get the whole amount of venom contained in the venom vesicle of the bee.

As far as your tablets are concerned, they are kept in perfect order, but I was unable to obtain permission for tests from the Institute for Rheumatic Diseases. I still hope that your wish will be fulfilled in 1961.

Accept, my esteemed colleague, my best wishes of good health and creative achievements.

Your N. YORISH.

Moscow 20 /IV 1961

The following is excerpted from *Bees and Health* by Professor N. P. Yorish, Moscow, U.S.S.R.:

METHODS OF OBTAINING BEE VENOM

The supply of venom of a working bee gradually increases during the first 2 weeks of its life, when it achieves a maximum, later the venom glands undergo a slow regression.

According to F. Fleury venom is obtained by subjecting bees to narcosis in a clean glass jar covered with a filter soaked in ether. Bees eject venom before they are narcotized. The jars are rinsed with water, which is then filtered and evaporated. The leftover substance is dry bee venom. The bees are dried in the sun, or in a warm place and returned to their hives. But it is not easy to get pure apitoxin by this method, and besides the bees do not give up all their venom and part of the bees perish.

B. Bek (1935) proposed to fill a glass jar with a wide mouth with distilled water and to cover this opening with a dry animal membrane—for instance, ox-bladder, or as the Chinese doctor Fan-Chu suggested, a chicken crop.

The bee is held by pincers (or between the fingers) and it is made to sting the membrane. The bee sting penetrates the thin membrane and the venom is promptly dissolved in water.

There are other ways of obtaining bee venom, but bees are killed in the procedure.

We have constructed a portable apparatus for securing bee venom without harm to the bees. This apparatus consists of a big cardboard box; it is very easy to shake off into it from a honey comb, a few thousand bees at a time. From this dark box the bee prisoners can get out only through special narrow passages which are constructed in such a way that each bee has to leave drops of venom on specially arranged plates. Bees conserve their stings and their capacity to fulfill all their functions.

METHODS OF BEE VENOM TREATMENT

For bee venom treatment a bee is applied with the help of pincers to the patient's skin, the exact location is chosen according to a chart, the skin cleaned with soap and water (alcohol contraindicated). The bee is set free after the sting and flies away leaving in the skin its sting with its apparatus, which continues to contract during two or more hours, until the whole venom vesicle is empty. One can usually see the end of this contraction with the naked eye. Only then should the sting be extracted. The small wound may be treated with any indifferent ointment.

The following method may be used:

Days	*Number of stings*	*Days*	*Number of stings*
1	1 bee	6	6 bees
2	2 bees	7	7 bees
3	3 bees	8	8 bees
4	4 bees	9	9 bees
5	5 bees	10	10 bees

After this first period of treatment, that is after 55 bee stings, one should make a pause of 3-4 days and continue the treatment applying 3 bees daily. During this second course (about 1½ months) the patient should receive venom from about 140-150 bees, that is 180-200 bee stings through the whole treatment.

Patients who spend their vacation in a house of rest or in a sanatorium can receive apitoxinotherapy according to the following chart:

Days	*Number of bee stings*
1	2 bees
2	4 bees
3	6 bees
4	8 bees
5	9 bees

From the 6th to the 24th day the patient is given 9 bee stings daily.

If after the two courses of treatment the patient is not cured, and shows no marked improvement, the treatment should be discontinued.

APPARATUS FOR APITOXINOTHERAPY (resumé)

It is usually difficult to catch a bee, without being stung. Bees caught with the help of the usual pincers eject venom if the slightest pressure is exerted.

The author proposes an apparatus consisting of a portable box where bees can live several days and of special tweezers. The box may contain up to 100 bees, it is warm and there is enough air and food (syrup or honey). The box has two removable compartments, which can be refilled with food without disturbing the bees. To catch a bee one opens a side window, and when the bee crawls out it is easy to catch her with special pincers.

An improved model contains a piece of honey comb, which can be filled with honey or thick syrup. In this miniature bee hive bees can live a month or longer. During warm weather it can be installed near a window, and the bees allowed to hunt for nectar during the day, they will return in the evening.

The specially constructed tweezers make it possible to apply the bee to the patient's skin, to press all the venom out immediately after the patient is stung, and to extract the sting with its whole apparatus.

METHODS OF APITOXINOTHERAPY

A method of apitoxinotherapy by intracutaneous injections of apitoxin has been developed, it can be used in hospitals and clinics. This method makes precise doses and a strictly individual approach possible. Apitoxin, dissolved in distilled water or physiologic salt solution is introduced intracutaneously in small doses (c.1, 0.2, 0.3 mgs.).

Ionotherapy or electroionotherapy is a method by which

one introduces drugs through the undamaged skin with the help of continuous current. This method can be used in any medical institution which has the necessary equipment. Introduction of apitoxin by this method is devoid of unpleasant sensations—there is only a slight hyperemia of the part of the skin which has been subjected to ionophoresis.

Recently a method of apitoxinotherapy by inhalation has been devised.

A healthy person can easily stand 1-5 and even 10 simultaneous bee stings. They provoke only reddening of the skin, swelling, and burning sensations; 200-300 simultaneous stings result in poisoning (dyspnoea, cyanosis, tachycardia and convulsions), 500 simultaneous bee stings are deadly. There are people, however, who show increased sensitivity to bee venom; a single sting provokes general malaise, sharp headache, urticaria, vomiting and diarrhea.

Most people adapt themselves quickly to bee stings and show no reaction. Beekeepers who work with bees for many years can stand them without harmful reactions. Our statistics show that 74% of beekeepers acquire immunity during the first 3 years, 13% in the course of 10 years and 2% enjoy apparently congenital immunity.

Bee venom therapy is contraindicated in certain diseases as tuberculosis, arteriosclerosis, venereal diseases, etc.

TREATMENT OF BEE STINGS

We have proposed the following method (which has been approved by the Pharmacological Committee of the Scientific Medical Counsel of the Ministry of Public Health in the USSR). The bee sting and the attached venom glands should be extracted by special tweezers and a special ointment containing calendula and alcohol applied locally.

A special first aid box contains pincers, ointment, a glass applicator, instructions and a small mirror, for face and neck stings.

In serious cases of bee poisoning bed rest is indicated, 50-

100 gr. of 40% alcohol per oz. is effective. It is still better to give the patient a solution of honey in 40% alcohol (about 20 gr. of honey to 200 gr. of alcohol) 25-50 gr. at one time. A honey and vitamins drink is also recommended. 100 gr. of honey and 500 mgr. of Vitamin C are dissolved in warm boiled water, the solution is to be kept in a cool place and the patient is to be given ½ glass of it every hour.

Cold moist dressings or dressings of boric solution (1 teaspoon to 1 glass of water) are applied locally. If necessary heart stimulants, sedatives or sleeping pills may be given.

Stings in the eye are very dangerous, because of a possible damage to the eyeball. The patient must be placed under the care of an eye specialist immediately.

On the Therapeutic Use of the Products of Apiculture

by Dr. N. P. Yorish

Folk medicine calls bee venom curative poison, and not without reason. After having passed the test of time, it has now passed the thresholds of hospitals. Thousands of persons afflicted with rheumatism, neuritis, hypertension and other diseases have regained their health, and taken their place in life, thanks to the outstanding therapeutic qualities of bee venom. Bee venom is a powerful antibacterial substance. A component of bee venom, histamin, lowers the blood-pressure in such concentrations as 1:250,000,000 and even 1:500,000,000. Bee venom does not lose its therapeutic properties by freezing, or by heating up to 100 during 10 days, it is not affected by exposure to solutions of caustic alkali, or sulphuric acid, for 24 hours.

In the course of the last two decades, both in the Soviet Union and abroad, sufficient data have been collected about the therapeutic use of bee venom. Apitoxinotherapy has been used in rheumatic diseases: polyarthritis, myositis, carditis rheumatica (rheumatism of the heart), encephalitis rheumatica, iritis; in diseases of the peripheral nerves, inflammations of n. facialis, ischiadicus, femoralis etc.; in radiculitis, inflammation of the spinal nerve roots; in Basedow's disease and hypertension. In all these diseases a positive therapeutic effect can be achieved in most cases by a correct use of apitoxinotherapy. Bee venom treatment is contraindicated in tuberculosis of the lungs and bones, venereal and mental diseases, in decompensated cardio-vascular patients, in kidney diseases (nephritis, nephroso-nephritis), hepatitis, cholecystitis, and in diabetes melitus, diabetes insipidus, and other endocrine diseases.

As a medicament bee venom has many advantages. One should mention first of all its quick action on the organism, and the great difference between therapeutic, toxic and lethal doses. The toxic dose is much more than tenfold (the therapeutic) and the lethal dose a few hundred times larger than the therapeutic dose. At the same time, bee venom is a strong poison and physicians should check the possible susceptibility of the patient. This is the reason why, in working out our scheme of apitoxinotherapy, we always considered, and still consider of utmost important, the location of the bee sting. That is, the exact place on the body where the bee is applied to the skin. On this depends not only the reaction of the organism, but the action of the venom itself, which may lead to fatal consequences for the patient. Experience shows that bee stings in the eye ball, even through the eyelid, in the soft palate, lips, nose, neck, temporal region, sexual organs, etc., might be very dangerous, and even cause the death of the patient. It is well known that bee venom is a poison with a general toxic action—that it affects all organs and systems; that is, the organism as a whole.

In the course of the last few years, we were able to observe the therapeutic effect of bee venom on brucellosis. And at the present time one of the Ural clinics uses bee venom treatment of brucellosis under hospital conditions. It is true, that in this severe illness, it is sometimes necessary to repeat the treatment (200 bee stings) 2, 3, or even 4 times.

During these last years apitoxinotherapy has been used in a great extent in the Soviet Union and other states of the people's democracy. Preparations, such as Virapin (Czechoslovakia) and Apisartron (East Germany) are widely used. But clinical observations in Roumania, Dr. Alexander Parteniu—in China, Dr. Fan-Chu and others—and in the U.S.S.R., Artemov, Kireev, Gusev, Yorish and others—show that natural bee venom, introduced by the sting of the bee is still more effective. At the same time, experience shows that it is extremely difficutl to grasp the bee by its wings, or thorax, and to avoid being stung. Catching a bee with the usual anatomical pincers is not a good method either, because the slightest pressure may provoke the secretion of venom, and this may happen much sooner than one is able to apply the bee to the patient's skin. Therefore we recommend the use of pincers "1-59" which we have devised: these are anatomical pincers of the usual kind, but with their free ends standing 3 mm. apart. This allows us to grasp the bee delicately by the thorax, and to put it on the patient's skin. Young bees, which have very little venom stored, cannot be held by these pincers. The pincers have two small metallic plates affixed to it, which enable us to pull out the sting with all the structures attached, right after the patient has been stung, but, naturally, after the whole venom from the poison bag has been absorbed by the skin capillaries. This is very important, because many patients have to wait an hour or longer, until the sting apparatus of the bee, which has an autonomous nervous system, finally ceases to contract. It is also required by physicians, who use the bee sting method of bee venom therapy according to "Temporary Instruction for Apitherapy: treatment by stings of living bees," which has been approved by the Bureau of the Presidium of the Scientific Committee of the Ministry of Public Health of the USSR, May 10, 1957. It is obvious that the pincers "1-59," are not only a time saving device for the patient, but that their use gives us the necessary guarantee that all the venom of the bee is left in the skin. This universal pincers can be made to order by any skilled locksmith, or anatomical pincers can be easily adapted for the purpose.

Bee Venom Preparation "Melassin" as a Remedy and Disease-Preventing Agent

by L. F. KONONENKO

Docent, Director of the Nervous Diseases Clinic, Faculty of Pediatrics, Institute of Medicine, Kharkov, U.S.S.R.

The bee venom preparation "melassin" produced in our Institute has proved to be a highly effective remedy and disease-preventing agent. An all-round study of its chemical and physical properties showed that it contains many trace elements. With the aid of chromatography we discovered in the bee venom the presence of 14 free amino acids. We also detected the essence of the "Langer's base" to which some authors attributed the basic effect of bee venom: it is "coniine," an alkaloid. The colorimetric method and biological tests helped in detecting steroid substances with androgenic and corticoidal activity, whose presence was corroborated by experimental and clinical observations. Desoxyribonucleic and ribonucleic acids and hyaluronidase have also been found in the preparation. The melassin preparation is not toxic, possesses no cumulative properties and produces no side effects. This has been confirmed on cold- and warm-blooded animals which were administered in various ways different doses of the preparation in acute and chronic experiments.

Experiments and clinical observations showed that melassin exerts good anti-inflammatory, depressory and anaesthetic action, improves oxidation processes and trophic function and also aids in regulating the hormonal function of the organism.

The preparation proved active in case of experimental infection of guinea pigs with diphtheria, giving a distinct anti-necrotic effect. A study of melassin in cases of experimental artherosclerosis in rabbits showed its influence in reversing the course of the disease.

Hypotensive properties of melassin have been confirmed in experiments on dogs suffering from centrogenous hypertonia and on rabbits with reflex hypertonia and also on cats, in some acute cases of this disease.

The therapeutic effects of the preparation were studied on experimental theophyline-adrenalin myocarditis in rabbits and confirmed by electrocardiograms and pathohistological data. Experiments with isolated rabbit intestines proved that melassin affects the contractive function of unstriated muscles, thus making it possible to use the preparation in anesthesia and to accelerate the uterine contractions during childbirth.

The high therapeutic activity of the preparation has been corroborated by electrocardiography (1,800 tests before and after treatment), ballistocardiography, arteropiezographs and oxyhemometry, platysmography and biochemical analysis (electrophoresis on paper of protein fractions of blood serum, cholesterine, potassium, calcium).

Electrocardiography showed that in most of the patients the frequency of heart beats drops by 5-25 beats per minute, the intra-auricular and intra-ventricular conductivity is improved and the systolic function normalized.

Clinical experiments and observations (on 1,689 patients) throw light on the mechanism of the therapeutic action of the preparation and made it possible to recommend its wide application for the treatment of cardiovascular diseases (hypertonia, atherosclerosis, coronary deficiency, hypertonic crises, obliterating endarteritis), acute and chronic cases of rheumatism, non-specific polyarthritis, diseases of the peripheral nervous system, etc. Treatment may be given both in hospitals and out-patient clinics.

APPENDIX F

The Dora Garrod-Thomas Trust

For Rheumatic Research

LETTERS SHOULD BE ADDRESSED TO:
The Secretary
The Dora Garrod-Thomas Trust
c/o Messrs. Merrimans
3 & 4 Lincolns Inn Fields
London, W.C. 2

20th October, 1952

Dr. Joseph Broadman,
Cumberland Hotel,
Marble Arch, W. 1

DEAR MR. BROADMAN,

On the eve of your leaving for New York I wish to put on record, on behalf of this Trust, our great appreciation of your selfless and public-spirited action in coming to this country at your own expense and on your own initiative for the sole and specific purpose of surveying the practice and application of Dr. G. Laughton-Scott's method of treatment for non-rheumatoid rheumatism. It is a matter of great gratification to the Trust and to Dr. Laughton-Scott that you have expressed your strong interest in his work in this way and it is the chief purpose of this letter to record the association we have made together for the further dissemination in America of the knowledge which has been achieved here.

As you are now, I think, satisfied that Dr. G. Laughton-Scott has developed a method of treatment for fibrositis and similar complaints which is probably more efficacious than any of the present known remedies, we shall be glad if you will do what you can to get this knowledge accepted in America. In particular, we have agreed with you that we will try and get some influential persons or bodies to set up clinics, either for industrial cases or for general ones, similar to those which have been started in this country.

As you have stated your willingness to serve in this way, we would be greatly obliged to you if you would consider yourself as generally representing our interests for the purpose noted above in the U.S.A. We are gratified that you have already offered to donate your services for the organization and furtherance of efforts in the way suggested.

You are aware that it is quite impossible for us to provide the dollars for financing free or assisted clinics for demonstration purposes in the U.S.A. We feel sure, however, that as soon as the importance of this treatment for rheumatic complaints becomes recognized in America—and this sort of knowledge usually does not take long to be appreciated in your country—the necessary funds will be forthcoming there. We will always be glad to contribute apparatus, and I know that Dr. Laughton-Scott will place his services at your disposal for demonstrations in New York, if these can be arranged.

We know that you will do what you can in the cause of relieving suffering from rheumatic complaints that fall under our area of attack, and it remains only to wish you success in your efforts in America and bon voyage on your journey home.

With kind regards,
Yours sincerely,
(signed) N. GARROD-THOMAS

My late sister's trust has a very warm corner in my heart, and this makes me doubly sorry that I am unable to meet you before your return to thank you personally for your interest in Scott's work, and the very practical way in which you have shown your interest.

(signed) N. GARROD-THOMAS

Author's comment: On their part, these people were ready to extend all the help which the laws of that time allowed.

Had we been able to secure the additional needed cooperation and support essential for bringing the Scott method here on a larger scale, it is plain to see that many more Americans would have been benefited by now.

APPENDIX G

Dr. Bodog F. Beck's Letter to Dr. Edithe E. Nichols

Nov. 23, 1938

MY DEAR DR. NICHOLS:

The present writing as you may surmise, is motivated by your article entitled—"Rheumatoid Arthritis, Treatment With the Sting of the Honey-Bee," which appeared in the September 15th, 1938, issue of the New York State Journal of Medicine. At first, I intended to ignore the matter entirely but my mail is heaped every day with so many protests against the article and with reproaches for my "doing nothing about the affair" that I finally had to yield.

You very well know my interest in the therapy and you will easily comprehend not only my disappointment but also my surprise when you stated in your summary that "Bee Sting Therapy had no constant or noteworthy effect in the treatment of rheumatoid arthritis. The results were so discouraging that we felt we were not justified in continuing this form of treatment." I fully realize that the "we" is not a *pluralis modestiae* but *pluralis majesticus*—which of course included the department of Medicine of Cornell University College.

To refresh your memory, may I quote from your letter, dated September 10, 1937—"I would like very much to see you to talk to you about some of the problems we encounter in the treatment of arthritis." You must have accorded to me some competence in the field. I was glad to accept the invitation for the date you suggested, Wednesday, September 6th at 2 o'clock, because, as you wrote, you had no clinic yourself on that day and you would have more time to talk over matters with me.

As you remember, I called at the New York Hospital on the date mentioned above and so far as I can recall, spent over an hour discussing various phases of Apitherapy, which as you acknowledged and I could see myself, were entirely new to you.

Maybe you will also remember that the first question I asked was whether you had obtained results with the Bee Venom. My inquiry, of course referred to both the injectable Bee Venom and to live bees. You frankly admitted that you had no success with either method. After further discussion I made you understand that both the dosage you administered was insufficient and that also the intervals were too far apart that under the circumstances you could not obtain any results. I well recall the severe case of arthritis of a man in the ward whom you showed to me, who was supposed to have gotten one-tenth of a cc. Apicosan a week before, two-tenths of a cc. the same week and was expected to have three-tenths the following week, etc. That dose could not be more helpful to him that it would be to try to extinguish a blazing fire in a huge warehouse with a medicine dropper.

I suggested, in a most friendly spirit, to call any time at my office and I assured you that you were more than welcome to all my experience which it took me many tedious years to acquire. Besides, as you remember, I offered to treat any patient you might refer to me with the understanding that there would be no charge for any services. You promised to send me some difficult cases so that I could convince you of the efficacy of the therapy. I was not only frightened but was highly delighted to have an opportunity to win you over to the cause.

You were good enough, however, to accept my invitation to call at my office with some member of your medical staff and Emil Greider, the Patterson bookkeeper who assisted you. Maybe you will also remember that I demonstrated in my office the method on several cases especially on one arthritic deformans case, on which I applied sixty-five stings in your presence. Possibly you will also recollect that you recognized, among the fifteen or twenty waiting patients in my office, some patients who had visited at the New York Hospital, your own clinic, for several months without any benefits. You interviewed them and they all reported to you how much they had improved under my treatment in a short time. My secretary overheard the conversation (I purposely left you alone with them) and I can assure you that nobody was more shocked at your report in the New York State Journal of Medicine than this same secretary who knows all about my work and its results. I never heard from you again until I came across your article.

May I add here that from most of the forty or fifty cases I treated daily in my office, I did not receive any compensation whatsoever because I am preparing to submit a report soon of many thousands of severe cases to try to convince the medical profession that the treatment with live bee stings is so far not only the best, but the only, successful cure (not only treatment) for the so-called incurable and hopeless arthritics. As you can see, we utterly disagree.

Of course, your damnatory report, so utterly unauthentic, being backed up by the reputation of Cornell University, aroused considerable attention; the daily papers and the radio, spread it all over the United States in 24 hours. I do not expect that my so far over 2,000 cured cases will have such a favorable assignment. But this is the irony of fate, you are sitting soft in an institution supported by a foundation of 20 million or more while I must pay for all the humanitarian services from my own pocket. My faith in truth is my consolation. The widely publicized article in the paid press, however, that your scientific research (carried out with the utmost care) decided "once and for all" the uselessness of treatment with live bees is not final by any means. As I said, I have faith that fair play will triumph in the end.

It is rather curious that the medical profession, for ages, have opposed progress. You know the story of the other Hungarian fanatic, Dr. Semelweiss, who was bold enough to blame the physicians to be the cause of puerperal sepsis because they attended to confinements without washing their hands after autopsies, and thus became the father of Antisepsis. He reduced the mortality from 26% to ½% in his own department, yet, was hounded by the profession until he died in an insane asylum. Germs were not accepted those days, but today even arthritis is treated with the aid of them. Everything is germs today. How things change.

There ought to be an 11th commandment that people would not write on subjects that they do not understand. An article appeared recently in another eminent publication where a doctor branded the method with live bees impractical because bees cannot be used during the winter months. Another false statement. I would like to give the doctor, right on the middle of his nose, during sub-zero weather only one single sting. The virulence undoubtedly decreases during the winter, but plenty of it is left. If you read the "Chemiker Zeitung" 1938, Vol. 73, p. 637, you will see my statement confirmed. The bee generates the venom during the first 15 days of its life and during that time the virulence increases, reaching on the 15th day its maximum potency. After that, the venom glands almost entirely degenerate but the venom in the bag remains active until the end of the bee's life. This is the wisdom of nature. One filled bag will suffice for the entire life of the bee, because if she uses it once, there is no need of it any more. One cannot expect, of course, that the average doctor should know that—but why make incorrect statements?

Handling live bees, and knowing all about them, is unfortunately not very easy. Your case also proves it, because after 18 months you still had to engage a Beekeeper to apply the bees. I would have gladly made an expert out of you in several lessons as I did with innumerable other physicians. The Beekeeper will not do it. Why lose his livelihood? Just last Sunday, November 20th, a doctor spent the entire day with me (name and address gladly furnished on request) getting instructions, of course, without charge for them. So far he had 100 cured cases with live stings and called the treatment the greatest boon for arthritis. The bees were supplied to him by a beekeeper and were supposedly "special medical bees." He had to pay a very high price for them. I told him to order them from the A. I. Root Co., Medina, Ohio, and he can get about 10,000 of the same medical bees for $2.50.

There are plenty of difficulties with this method but it can be learned. A professional man, especially in the big cities, will have some obstacles which, however, can be easily overcome. You ask Dr. Carl A. Zoll of the Wickersham Hospital. After he visited me several times, he installed a hive of bees in his office and today uses daily a good many hundreds. His results are also excellent, like those of many others.

So far you are the only one who has condemned the method.

You will probably wonder what my real purpose is in writing you this letter. Permit me to remark right here that your method of applying the bees and the intervals of their administration, in spite of the fact that I called your attention to errors in technic, at the same time you commenced the treatments, are still entirely defective. I will explain later on what I mean. The 27 cases you selected did not justify you in condemning the treatment.

You admit in your article that you had selected severe cases which had previously received various forms of treatment without beneficial results. The duration of the ailments in themselves, among them one of 30, one of 10, 2 of 9, 2 of 8, one of 6, 4 of 5 years etc., is positively unfair, especially for one who had not had previous experience. The same applies to the selection of cases with regard to ages: 60-8, 65, 58, 55 years etc. NOTE: In your experience with Apicosan, you carefully selected many mild cases in which the duration of the illness ranged only from 3 weeks, and in 36 cases, to one year or less. The partiality is very evident.

The manner alone, in which you computed your statistics is entirely objectionable. You admit that you obtained out of 27 cases, 3 marked improvement. This alone would not entitle you, yet, to denounce the method. There would be 24 cases left. You also admit 5 slight improvements which again does not warrant passing condemnatory sentence. Only 19 cases now remain for your statistical data. Two disliked the treatment after receiving 3 and 7 stings respectively, leaving only 17 cases. Out of the remaining 17, you discontinued the treatments in 12 cases because 5 suffered severe general or local reactions after receiving 24, 17, 14, 11 and 4 stings. The next 7 cases were discontinued because they became worse. In brief, there were hardly any cases left which would justify you to make such a broad and momentous statement. The absurdity of the article is astounding and has all the earmarks, that, it had for its main purpose, the sales argument—Apicosan vs. Bee-stings. Very scientific. . . .

The manifestation of the local and general reactions, I always consider a welcome symptom and no reason for discontinuing the treatments, just the contrary. Referring to the other few remaining cases, which became worse, I have never seen a patient yet who did not become worse during the treatment. Very often, patients feel pain in joints where they never felt any before but all pain gradually disappears. I usually explain this to my patients, and they are not only not afraid of the reactions, but are impatiently waiting for them. You cannot obtain improvement without reactions, and, the more severe the reactions, the greater the improvement. I feel authorized to make the statement, and not after only 27 cases either.

I cannot go into details in discussing the various phases of the reactions. All I do say, at the present time, is that though there is systematic and gradual immunization, I notice severe local and general reactions, they, however, disappear in 24 to 48 hours. What happened to your case which was confined in bed for 3 months, I am unable to say, but I can assure you that in well over two thousand cases which I have treated, I have never had a single case in which the general reaction lasted longer than 48 hours. The local reaction may persist for a longer time but it is always followed by a correspondingly, and often surprising, improvement.

You will permit me to call your attention, and I feel fully justified in doing so, to the fact that your procedure in many other respects was entirely wrong. To administer the stings once a week proves that you are not conversant with the entire principle. One must slowly and gradually immunize patients and they often require daily applications, or at one and two day intervals. That is, as soon as the former reactions are almost subsiding, the next ones must be applied. Your weekly administration, that is too long an interval, not only did you *not immunize* the patient, but *sensitized* him.

This explains your extremely severe reactions even after a few stings which forced you to give up further treatments in such cases. If you read the 3rd paragraph on page 101, of my book, "Bee Venom Therapy" you will understand what I mean. According to Dr. Gideon H. Wells, our most eminent pathological chemist, smaller doses are more effective to produce sensitization. He succeeded in sensitizing guinea pigs with a single dose of albumin as small as one twenty-millionth of a gram. Please do not overlook the fact that bees always inject some protein (pollen) with their venom and your beekeeper may have occasionally brought you bees to which different pollen was attached. You must know your bees, your venom . . . and also your onions. I frequently apply 100 stings on one patient without obtaining even slight or general reaction and two days later they come, smiling and happy, for 100 more. The matter is not as simple as it looks.

Your method of decreasing your weekly stings or discontinuing the treatments if any itching or general reactions manifested themselves, was also absolutely wrong. If you had increased the number of stings during consecutive treatment, there would have been no itching and less general reaction. The weekly intervals, however, did most of the mischief, but possibly Mr. Grieder could only come once a week.

It is not surprising that you had to drag out the treatments in some cases to 18, 15, or 14 months. I could show you very severe arthritis Deformans cases of seven and ten years standing, totally crippled, wandering from one institution to another and discharged as hopeless cases, who in three months after treatment with live stings, are able to get back to work. If you are interested, I will be only too glad to introduce them to you.

It is too bad that you did not accept my invitation to visit my clinic occasionally, instead of trying to administer such a severe blow to the increasing popularity of the treatment. Please understand that I do not feel a personal offense, but we must not forget that there are about 10 million arthritics in the U.S. who are anxiously awaiting their salvation. If you could read my correspondence from all over the U.S., Canada and also from Australia and Africa, it would astound you.

It is needless to say that I am quite distressed about the publicity in the daily papers and the talks over the radio which the condemnation of the method by Cornell University aroused. I do not accuse you of initiating this campaign, but it was certainly widely broadcast all over the country. I cannot tell you what resentment it caused among my patients who were restituted to health after many years of suffering. They object to your statement that the treatments were not worth the pain they caused.

One comment refers to you as the "Hen Medico" with her "completely cock-eyed" statistics. A colleague sarcastically remarked, that it was too bad you did not have a couple of fatal cases among the 27, because, by reporting them in addition to the case of the woman who was confined to bed for three months, it would have been very subservient to the cause of "Apicosan vs. Bee Stings. Many offer their services to confute your allegations and make it public. I am not in favor of such tactics. The work is too sacred to me.

It is also strange, that the article in the January, 1938, issue of "Annals of Internal Medicine" was also signed by you. In that article you reported 73% improvements with Apicosan and that you were "impressed with the definite improvement in the large percentage of patients" and that Apicosan was worthy of consideration.

On the other hand, in the article in the N.Y. State Journal of Medicine, your results with live bees were so discouraging that you did not feel justified in continuing this form of treatment. I thought that Apicosan was supposed to be made out of bee venom? If so, why this contradiction? Many physicians, of whom I succeeded in making converts, took the strongest exception to the conspicuous manner in which Apicosan (always in Italics and caps) was frequently mentioned in your article, giving even the name and address of the agent. One physician even sarcastically remarked, that it was too bad that the telephone number was not inserted and also several order slips for Apicosan.

They all consider such advertising unworthy of a high type institution like the Cornell University College. Between us, in perfect confidence, I can assure you that after many years of experience with several other types of injectable bee venom I find several others far superior to Apicosan. If you would have made a chemical analysis of Apicosan your attitude toward the product, I am certain, would have been different. Possibly you read in the "Medical Clinics" of North America, 1947, issue (p. 1617) an article entitled "The Arthritis Problem" in which Dr. Snyder of the Hospital for Ruptured and Crippled remarked that "with bee stings, they noted an (undeniable) improvement in several cases which had been very resistant to every other form of treatment. But the result with Apicosan in our clinic has so far been unsatisfactory."

The circulars sent out by the Kretschmar firm, immediately after the publication of your last article, Apicosan vs. Bee-stings, referring to your high praise of Apicosan and the condemnation of live bee stings, was positively distasteful. The printer's ink of your article was not even dry when this circular was "expressed" to the

150,000 physicians in the U.S. Don't you smell something, somewhere?

This letter is not written for the purpose of criticising your work or defending the treatment with live bee stings. This will be done in due course of time and not in the daily press either. I would not copy the privileges of an erudite University. The main purpose of my missive is to offer my services again and purely from a humanitarian standpoint. If you wish to assist me in a similar spirit, I would ask you to send me any or all of the cases in which you do not obtain results, with a repeated understanding that no fees of any kind will be accepted for the treatments. Do you consider this fair? I fully realize, that it may be rather difficult for you to comply exactly with my request because such patients, after having been badly burned, may be unwilling to submit again to the same treatment. But possibly you will be able to select some similar bad cases. I know you are in a position to do so.

Luckily poor Dr. Terc is dead and could not read your article. What would he have said to the statement (p. 1220) "that some of your patients improved from bee stings in their physical condition and sense of well being, but you considered it possibly due to the dramatic (comedy perhaps) nature of this form of therapy, because the administration of the stings is rather spectacular." You know that Dr. Terc used the treatment for 40 years, administered to the patient 150 to 200 stings on the same day, cured 82% of his cases, and claimed that there is not an arthritic case that could not be cured, with bee stings.

Please pardon me for some of my remarks which may seem to you objectionable, but be assured that they are dictated by a feeling of truth and fairness. I sincerely hope that with your kind cooperation we may still straighten out matters in the interest of this very noble and worth while cause.

Very sincerely yours,
BODOG F. BECK, M.D.

P.S. Too bad you wasted the good alcohol of the hospital washing the skin of the applicants before the application of the stings. I applied, the Lord knows how many, hundreds of thousands of stings without disinfecting the skin and frankly I have never seen a single infection. The venom itself will disinfect, besides, nothing destroys the venom quicker than alcohol, even if you "let it dry." The pollen, however, as your cases show, remains active.

APPENDIX H

Lecture by Dr. Terc in the Monthly Assembly of Beekeepers—February 11, 1904

Many years ago when I came to the conclusion that bee venom and its tremendous healing potential was one of the greatest importance as a means of treating rheumatism, I promised myself never—and under no conditions—to make these facts known to other than doctors or to have them published anywhere else than in medical journals.

I have kept true to this promise up to now. Owing to the fact, however, that I met with nothing but rebuffs from my medical colleagues so far, and spurned by the fear that my painstakingly acquired knowledge may sink into oblivion without ever gaining any attention, I followed your call hoping that you, my fellow beekeepers, might grant me some help in the interest of beekeeping in general and, in particular, support me in your own way in my endeavors of nearly 25 years.

In order to bring on a better understanding from your side of what I am going to say, I have to describe first the effect of bee venom on the healthy organism, and in doing so, might have to mention facts which are already known to you.

If a bee inserts her sting into the deeper layers of the skin, the poison gland deposits its contents simultaneously into it and there will occur, sometimes, a small deposit of blood around the place where the sting was inserted, but you will always find a swelling around the site of the sting, which first we call a wheal. This wheal eventually produces a swelling which may last as long as 2 or 3 days and which, in the beginning, causes a burning feeling that eventually subsides into itching and still later totally disappears. This wheal I mentioned is the permanent associate of a sting and I call this wheal the primary reaction. In persons sensitive to bee venom, we sometimes see reactions such as nausea, feeling of being in bad health and dizziness. These nervous reactions plus the swelling that follows the wheal, I call the secondary reaction of the body to the bee venom.

There are a very few healthy people who are inclined to faint when stung by a bee, but recover again in a very short time. I, myself, met such a person only once, but have heard of two ardent beekeepers in Germany who had to protect themselves carefully from being stung.

If persons subjected to serious diseases of the heart, such as degeneration of the large blood vessels (arteries) connected with a weakness of the heart, as well as persons who are likely to die in consequence of any excitement of any nature, are stung by bees, they may die as a consequence of these stings, but such cases would represent only the occasion and not the cause of death. An autopsy in such cases would reveal the true cause.

It can't be denied that bee stings under normal conditions may become dangerous and even deadly. That only happens, however, when healthy persons, unaccustomed to bee stings, are suddenly stung by a great number of bees. The great majority of human beings get gradually accustomed to bee venom. The more often they get stung, the less they will swell. Any nausea that may occur also decreases and finally ceases completely, as do the swellings. They have become immunized.

This immunity lasts over a limited time; at the beginning, perhaps only through one winter. If it has been acquired repeatedly for some consecutive years then it can be considered as permanent, or at least for the span of a few years.

There are, beyond any doubt, people that do not swell after having been stung by bees. That means that they have been born immune against bee venom. Such persons, in my opinion, are also naturally immune against rheumatism.

When first I read in various magazines that bee stings were a remedy against "rheumatism and gout" (incidentally, two totally different diseases), I smiled with pity about such statements written in a dilettantory way by laymen and empyrics [sic] in just the same way that my medical colleagues still laugh at me today—if they do not do worse than this. All the same I am convinced that mine is the glory for having established the peculiar relationship between bee venom and rheumatism and to have thrown some light on its efficacy in many ways and from all angles.

It was my own experience that induced me first to look into this matter seriously. When once mercilessly attacked by bees, my rather persistent and reoccurring muscular rheumatism never returned after this incident. From that time on, I took the risk to administer bee venom to people who suffered from rheumatism and even did not shy away from bribing poor people so as to gain experience with it.

Although I had achieved real success at this time, I was not able to get any real satisfaction out of the treatment because I had no actual insight into the mode of action of bee venom. This I was only able to understand in the course of treating the following case:

A lady who had suffered for years from deafness and head rheumatism in 1879 came to me for help because I, then, had acquired a reputation as a physican. The lady, who was very rich, had previously sought help from a great number of doctors and had used a lot of medications. She refused any and all of my suggestions in this line and also likewise declared every treatment I could think of as "of no use." "I had expected some new approach—that's why I came to see you," she told me. At that point, I remembered the bee stings and suggested that she should try this treatment, secretly hoping that she be discouraged, by telling her about the swellings, etc., she would have to expect, as she had become rather bothersome by refusing each and every previously made suggestion. She, however, willingly agreed to the proposition of having bee stings applied, as this was something she had not tried before. After that she came to me for treatment daily. She had no relief from her pains but on the other hand, showed no swellings whatsoever. When I mentioned to her that I doubted I could help her (at this point, she had 90 bee stings applied to her head), she insisted upon going on with the treatments. This morning, having increased the number of stings constantly, I applied 13 stings. The next morning I was told to come to her hotel. Her face was swollen to an alarming extent, her skin looked grey and she hardly could open her eyes. But, nevertheless, she was jubilant. "I am completely free of pain," she yelled, and "I have just heard the chime of the church bells."

The reluctance of any tendency to swell which I had expected to happen after such a long time, and its finally happening, simultaneously with a very obvious improvement in her rheumatic pains, convinced me more than ever of the peculiar connection that exists between rheumatism and bee venom.

From there on I gave my special attention to this connection with every new case of rheumatism that came my way. After many years of experience in this line without danger and without sacrifices for an ordinary physician, I found conclusively that people afflicted with true rheumatism do not swell when stung by bees; the number of stings needed to finally bring on a swelling, solely depends on the severity and previous duration of the disease. In light cases a few stings will prove to be sufficient. In severe cases, many hundreds or even thousands of stings may be needed until a swelling or secondary reaction can be achieved.

In very severe or in long established cases, I could observe a temporary ceasing of the first swellings which often lasted for days. After a few days, however, this secondary reaction reoccurred in a far more violent way than before. This happened repeatedly with various patients. As it is with non-afflicted persons who are of a nervous disposition, many suffer from violent general reactions such as nausea and even fainting attacks, so it can happen with rheumatically afflicted patients who, at this stage, may produce extremely violent reactions which will greatly perturb the patient himself as well as his relatives.

Even I was greatly disturbed by these symptoms which caused me many a painful hour of doubt and many sleepless nights before I had thoroughly studied them and then found them to be quite harmles. For years I have made it a rule to inform the patient and his family of all these symptoms in advance, and always emphasize the fact that these reactions were a favorable and crucial sign, which passes quickly and without causing any ill effects.

As known to every physician, there exists a number of pseudo-rheumatic diseases, that means ailments which show all the peculiarities of rheumatism but which are based on totally different causes and sometimes are even of a contagious nature. They can be immediately diagnosed by the instant, and most violent, reactions to bee venom. They are unfavorably influenced by bee venom and must under no circumstances be ever treated by it. There are, beyond doubt, some patients who will not tolerate bee venom although they are afflicted with a true rheumatism. We sometimes find a similar reaction in people who violently react aginst certain harmless and generally used medications, which can cause them great harm. (Idiosyncrasies.) In my very extensive practice, I have come across only one single case who would not tolerate bee venom.

Professor Lederer, in an article published in 1879 in the "Wiener Medizinishe Press" reports about such a case who reacted with extreme violence to the first bee sting he got. This, unfortunately, was Professor Lederer's first case he ever tried to treat with bee venom, and, thereafter, he lost any interest in this treatment because of this unfortunate experience. What is worse he discouraged all the other doctors from trying bee venom therapy by strongly influencing them through his article. I am more fortunate than he in this matter by coming across such a case only after I had seen a great number which followed the normal pattern. I was not influenced by this abnormal case in the least. There are exceptions to the rule everywhere.

Gentlemen: It would not be a difficult matter for me to prove to you, if you were physicians yourselves, what bee venom is able to do for rheumatic patients. If you were physicians, I could show you the histories of such cases. As it is, I do not want to bore you with facts which, necessarily, must be incomprehensible to you. I, therefore, give you only a short outline of some of the cases and refer you for further details to a paper on this subject which will be published very shortly.

Before I go into the description of the successes that can be achieved in the healing of the various forms of rheumatism, I want to stress the fact that every rheumatically afflicted patient has to be accustomed very gradually to bee venom. One should never apply more than 3 stings in one treatment at first. If the patient tolerates this quantity, one can gradually increase the daily amount of stings up to 100-150 without any fear. This statement shows clearly that, in cases of an acute rheumatism of the joints (rheumatic arthritis), one can not achieve quick results. As such results can be achieved by other remedies in a much quicker way, I always have tried to use those first. That does not say that I do not treat such cases with bee venom, but I have ceased to do so eventually for above mentioned reasons. I always have fallen back on bee venom in such cases where any other remedy was of no avail, where I came across relapses or when the heart was afflicted by a rheumatic disease, which unfortunately is so often the case.

In all such cases where I treated with bee venom from the beginning, no such heart afflictions ever developed or [else they] subsided during the treatment. In cases which I only saw at the advanced stage of rheumatic heart condition, it was not always possible to prevent or curb the development of a chronic heart disease (but which I have done successfully more often than not) so it was made possible at least, to compensate to this extent that the patient, when cured of rheumatism, felt as a perfectly healthy person without a heart affliction. These successes I treasure most because of the high mortality in rheumatic patients owing to a heart condition.

Years ago I was called to a patient who previously had been treated for rheumatism of the joints but completely without any success. This lady was not able to move in her bed, suffered in addition with a severe heart disease, and, having heard about bee venom, desperately wanted to try this treatment. After I had examined her very carefully and decided to take the risk, a relative of hers remarked, "Are you actually contemplating to torture this death-bound person?" I first applied one single sting, then after half an hour, two, and after another hour again, two more. She tolerated them well without hardly feeling any pains on application. I stayed for half a day with her to keep her under observation and finally felt entitled to promise her complete recovery.

The next day I showed her gardener, a beekeeper himself, how to apply the stings, and three weeks later the "death-bound" patient left her bed for the first time in years. Unfortunately the patient, immediately after having finished the cure, left the district without having achieved full immunization. At the last examination, however, she was not only completely cured of rheumatism but, at the same time, the previous murmur of her heart had entirely ceased.

Twelve years ago I was called to the bedside of a lady. She suffered some months with rheumatism of the joints, an affliction of the heart and a pronounced rise in temperature. As she could not tolerate any more drugs, she had decided on bee venom. After she had been given 600 stings, she was completely cured. Although she had suffered repeatedly from severe attacks of rheumatism before consulting me, she never had a reoccurrence of the disease during the following 10 years which I had occasion to see her from time to time, even though she exposed herself to all kinds of weather conditions.

Gentlemen: Although I do not want to tire you with all

sorts of case histories, I would like to mention one case which seems to me of extreme importance. The person in question was a lady in her early fifties who had suffered, before seeing me, from repeated attacks of muscular rheumatism plus rheumatism of the joints. At the time she consulted me, she had developed a rheumatic marasm combined with an inflammation of the valves of the heart and pericardium. The pain in many of her joints and especially the one in her heart, plus shortness of breath and high temperature, forced her to stay in bed permanently. She, too, could tolerate no more medications. A very carefully applied course of treatment with bee stings, extending through the summer, brought a complete cure of her disease. The murmur in her heart had practically ceased, the rheumatic pains had completely vanished, as had her shortness of breath. Her general condition was perfect. She had been given 2,000 stings.

Muscular rheumatism offers the most favorable field for the treatment with bee stings, the acute form and especially the chronic form of muscular rheumatism, regardless of its duration.

In 1879 I got in contact with one of the most interesting cases of this kind. In 1877 the patient in question had got over a severe attack of muscular rheumatism. Despite the most careful treatment given to him then, an affliction centered in the bicuspitalis of his heart. The joints and muscles of the base of his head were especially affected, which severely hampered the mobility of his head and his neck muscles and moreover made it difficult for him to breathe. The thorax was immobile and like an armor, his walk painful and dragging. The patient was in a very much rundown condition and tired of life.

When I suggested bee stings, he said: "Do what you like with me. I do not care. There is no hope left for me anyhow!" He, furthermore, said, "I might be a guinea pig as well." I gave him 1,000 bee stings during the first summer. In the fall, he went on long hikes. During the following winter, he took up skating again and felt very well. Because of slight relapses, he had to undergo two after treatments of 150 stings until he achieved a complete cure. He now stays completely healthy, is happily married and the father of several children. He holds an important position on the educational board.

Gentlemen: In this category of disease, I could mention a lot of cases, too, but will confine myself to one more. In 1883, a man 60 years old caught a severe cold by being coatless when driving his cart when he freely perspired. He fell the victim of a severe general muscular rheumatism as a consequence. The joints were not affected. I saw him first on August 12th. He had lost a great deal of weight, suffered from lack of appetite, had temperatures and sleepless nights owing to constant pain. He had lost all the strength of his hands, so much so that he could neither write nor hold a spoon. On top of all this, he was subject to spasms. At his advanced age and very poor general condition, the prognosis was not very much in his favor.

Despite all this and against my own and others' convictions, I tried bee stings. I proceeded very cautiously and—after 160 stings—was rewarded by the first swellings. After a further two weeks, the temperature subsided, sleep and appetite returned and the pains became bearable. Up to November 15th, I applied 1,000 more bee stings. The patient felt very well. The various remaining paralyses were treated with faradic treatment and so eliminated. The following year he got 100 more bee stings so as to maintain his immunity. The patient went on living for 25 years longer and kept free and immune of rheumatism.

The same results were achieved with chronic rheumatism which was, more or less, restricted to the joints. Out of the great number of such cases I treated and cured, I only want to mention a few. The following one belongs to one of my very first cases. A male patient, a railway locksmith, 29 years old, became critically ill, after he had suffered repeated attacks of rheumatism. In the beginning of May, 1879, he suffered a vehement inflammation of his knee joints on both sides. He became bedridden and was treated inside and outside of various hospitals without success.

On New Year's Day, I saw the patient in his basement flat for the first time. He looked pitiful, had lost a lot of weight, his temperature went up, alternately, with profuse sweating. Both knees, in consequence of exudates in the knee joints, were considerably swollen and very painful. Out of sheer pity, I started an immediate treatment despite the unfavorable time of the year, as he, a married man and father, was in danger of dismissal by the railway. I gave him up to January 17th, over 70 stings, without achieving any reaction and with only very poor results. Owing to extremely cold weather, I had to interrupt the treatment until March 6th. All other medication given in the meantime was of no avail, either.

From March 6th to the end of April, this man got an additional 250 stings. At this point, the first swellings made their appearance. At the end of April he could leave his bed for the first time for a short while. The treatment was continued until the end of May. On June 1st, he started to work again. The patient now came to my office when off duty and got 1,100 more stings for the sake of complete immunization (up to the end of November). In 1885, after a severe influenza, he suffered a rheumatic paricarditis, had 100 more bee stings and totally recovered without any relapses since then.

Gentlemen: I cannot spare you from hearing about the next case, because it refers to one of my severest cases and, by doing so, clearly shows what actually can be achieved by bee venom treatment.

The patient, a woman of 42, came to me in the beginning of August, 1886. She had been afflicted six years previous to calling on me and had looked in vain for help at various doctors and spas. She was the picture of utmost ill health, a mere skeleton. All her joints were severely swollen, thickened and deformed. Under great pain, she managed to move from her bed to a chair in order to spend another sleepless night, tortured with pain after returning to her bed. Here, too, sheer desperation was needed to commence a treatment at all.

Between the beginning of August and the beginning of October, she was given 1,700 stings. She left Marburg looking extremely well and free of pains. On her return in the following spring, she got 300 more bee stings, was completely cured and looked the picture of health. The previously crippled joints remained crippled, of course, but she could walk and remained perfectly free of pains and free of relapses up to the present date. The only regret she had was not to have turned to bee stings sooner.

The great progress in medicine throws much light upon the so-called "rheumatic diseases." The "deforming gout of the joints," now rheumatic arthritis, however, was put apart from all other actual rheumatic diseases. This rheumatic arthritis does not respond to any known remedies, and severe deformities and year-long diseases are the lot of such afflicted persons. Even this disease, however, can be cured by bee venom, provided one does not wait too long before the start of the treatment.

Not taking into consideration all the cases which I treated and kept under observation for years afterwards, I would like to mention a special case which is a typical example and which, I am sorry, up to this day was not presented at a clinic before starting to treat with bee venom. I might be laughed at today, but the future will rehabilitate me.

In February, 1900, a young female patient started to show some swellings at all joints of her fingers which, as she expressed it herself, looked like frostbites and were very painful. She had no temperature with it, whatsoever. Gradually all joints of her extremities were affected, even those at the base of her skull. Finally, she got afflicted with violent stabbing pains in her chest and shortage of breath. She was bedridden more and more frequently and, in the beginning of 1902, getting out into the open caused her violent pains and great difficulties.

All known ways of treatment, hot air included, had no effect on her at all.

She got in touch with me at the end of March, 1902, after

an affliction of over two years. The patient was anemic and emaciated, all joints of her extremities, especially those of the upper ones, were thickened and painful. The hand and middle hand joints were already characteristically turned upwards, she could not straighten her elbows anymore, and her knees contracted in spasm from time to time. She had an enormous exudate on the right side of her chest and her urine contained great quantities of albumin.

She got her first bee sting at the end of March. The first slight swellings occurred only after she had 300 bee stings. Then they ceased, only to reoccur again, which up and down lasted until November. She by then had had 5,600 bee stings. The relapses she suffered during the treatment became slighter and more insignificant all the time. For the benefit of total immunization, I continued to apply bee stings for weeks on end even after the attacks had completely ceased.

The albumin had completely vanished from her urine as early as June, the exudate practically ceased. At the end of September, the patient was completely free of pains, despite the "do or die" treatment she was receiving, and went walking for hours. She felt perfectly well. I drew her attention to the possibility of relapses and also to the necessity of a second cure. She stood the following winter well, although she got caught in the "Bora" in Trieste. She had a slight relapse in March, 1903, despite her looking extremely well, which subsided after very few bee stings.

During the following summer she was given 1,000 bee stings. Her general condition was excellent, besides the fact that at certain critical days each month, she sustained slight swellings of a few joints of her hands which subsided again by themselves after two or three days. This was only the proof of the patient's extraordinary great predestination toward rheumatism and the extreme stubbornness of the conquered disease. Her immunization will have to be renewed for years to come. This case is practically and theoretically of highest importance and interest.

Bee stings have proved themselves to be likewise efficacious in cases of a rheumatic affliction of the nerves, and I can quote a great number of successes in this field also. Needless to say that here, too, cases of long standing presented a greater problem than those treated in time. I use this opportunity to stress the fact that only purely rheumatic pains and inflammation of the nerves can be treated with bee stings but not ordinary neuralgias.

Having told you so much of my successes, I feel I owe you some unfavorable reports, too. Of an unusual and drastic treatment, one expects quick and drastic results. You have been told earlier that this can *not* be done with bee stings. That is the reason why so many patients lost their confidence if quick success could not be achieved in the treatment. It is a deplorable fact that the bad name the bee venom is linked with, is mostly created by these kind of patients. Other patients again stubbornly declare to be satisfied with the ceasing of their pains, and were not to be persuaded to allow themselves to be fully immunized. Relapses thus brought on by patients themselves, gave the cause for their opinion "Oh well, those bee stings are no good either." Other patients again got frightened by the finally achieved swellings and the following general strong reactions and never became disciples of this treatment. Only too many of the patients—right in the midst of their treatment—became persuaded by some adversary of the same, that it was no good. More so, even during the first years of my treatment, it was often I myself who, by sheer lack of experience, got discouraged in cases where I had too slow a progress—to continue the treatment without any assurance of success. I think I also should mention that I often tried to apply bee stings in too long neglected cases, too crippled cases or on cases that were already too poor in health.

I often got discouraged, hurt, had my very living threatened, and was on the verge of giving up. Yet today—after 25 years of relentless experiments—and being still in touch with a great number of my former rheumatic patients who are now completely cured after they had tried all other cures in vain before—without any effect, were slowly dying and driven into despair—I feel that I must go on by fulfilling my duty to humanity in constantly drawing the attention of all my colleagues to the treatment with bee venom.

All those patients who had been treated with other remedies without success or where other forms of treatment can't be applied any more, must be considered as suitable cases.

It, naturally, is up to the physician himself to choose the right treatment in specific cases. Moreover, the patient and the doctor should always keep in mind that bee venom eliminates the cause of the disease and thereby the disease itself, but is unable to make good the outer deformations and changes in joints which have been effected by nature previous to the treatment. Even here, however, an improvement can happen. It is important not to wait too long before using bee venom. I maintain that each case of rheumatism (exceptions I mentioned not included) *can be cured* by bee venom. I do not hesitate to declare most emphatically that by a treatment of rheumatism with bee stings in good time, all the disastrous diseases that go with it can be prevented. The future will show me correct.

The effect of bee venom is a local as well as a general one (which is proved by the immunization). If somebody maintains that the bee stings act only by effect on the skin, about in the same way as a Vesicator does, he talks about it like a blind man would talk about color. Now, having nearly come to the end of my lecture, I wish to mention the most interesting thing which I have saved up for this moment. Dr. Joseph Langer, Professor at the University of Prague, observed that in a solution of 0.10% of the effective properties of bee venom (which was made up by himself) certain microorganisms (which might be the cause of rheumatism) are barely able to exist and do not multiply. If transferred into a solution, favorable to their conditions of living, they start to grow and multiply again. Even though those tiny organisms did not perish in Langer's bee venom solution, it still must be said that the conditions in the human body are a vastly different proposition. In their exhausted state and rendered into a stage of vastly diminished resistance by bee venom, and moreover attacked by the oxygen of the body and so killed, the cause of rheumatism seems to be eliminated. In an organism that is made immune to bee venom, the tiny bacteria which have penetrated into the body become weakened immediately, and later on die.

Gentlemen: I have put your patience to a long test, and thank you for having given me your attention.

Concluding, I wish to express the hope that sometime in the future it will be recognized that bee venom is the really and truly specific remedy for rheumatism and that it will be possible to make the treatment painless by injecting either the serum of Langer or any other equivalent of an injectable bee venom. Nobody would be more delighted with such a development than me, who has done nothing more than to utilize a very ancient folk-medicine remedy in more than 500 cases over more than 25 years. I have studied its effects to such an extent that now, based on the knowledge acquired, it can be tried by any physician. For all the humiliations and hostilities I had to suffer through all those years and for all the sacrifices I willingly made, I would ask for only one reward: I would like to live long enough to see that the bee venom gets its full recognition and that beekeeping, thereby, finds a much wider field.

APPENDIX I

Letter from Dr. Hermann N. Sander to Dr. Broadman

Manchester, New Hampshire
November 21, 1961

DEAR DOCTOR BROADMAN:

During the past five years I have fully treated some—131 patients with various rheumatic diseases. These include 35 with bursitis of the shoulder or hip joints, 32 of which were completely relieved and have needed no further treatment; 27 rheumatoid arthritics of which 21 were completely or markedly relieved with 6 showing poor response; 46 cases of osteoarthritis, 36 of which had good to excellent response while 10 showed poor response; 16 cases of fibromyositis, 15 of which showed good to excellent response with 1 poor response; 1 Tic Doloureaux with excellent response; 2 cases of gout with good response; 2 cases of migraine with good response; 3 cases of Marie-Strumpel, 1 showing good response, 2 no response. This does not include some—100 or more cases who did not follow through with the treatment and whom I cannot include in this series.

The following reports are examples of cases successfully treated:

Mr. R. S., age 52, painful shoulder which was worse at night making it almost impossible to sleep for a period of about a year. This man had some limitation of motion on internal rotation and abduction but no particular point of tenderness. X-ray diagnosis was osteoarthritis of left shoulder. There was no evidence of calcification of the bursae. On April 13, 1959 he received his first treatment with bee venom (Forapin) showing no sensitivity to skin test. He was treated every other day with increasing doses, noticing his first improvement on the fifth treatment. On the eleventh treatment the next stronger solution of Forapin was started, gradually increasing the dose. On the fifteenth treatment a complete plaque was noticed. This dose was continued, being 2 cc. in amount, with which 25-30 wheals were made. The total number of treatments was twenty. The last six treatments resulted in complete plaques. This patient has been seen for other reasons since this treatment with no complaints, the last visit being November 13, 1961 for a physical checkup. He stated that at this time there had been no further pain in the shoulder and that he sleeps very well and is very happy with the results.

Mrs. J. W., age 49, bursitis right shoulder and frozen shoulder. This patient had a first attack of acute right subdeltoid bursitis in July, 1957, and was treated at her camp with immobilization and analgesics. The shoulder became almost fixed with marked limitation and abduction and internal rotation. She was started on Forapin three times a week, completing the first course on May 8, 1958. At this time she had about a 60% recovery as compared to when she was first seen by me on February 19, 1958 at which time she was limited to about 15 degrees abduction and about 75-80% impairment in internal rotation.

The treatment was augmented by some physical therapy. She was discharged for the summer and was seen the next time in February, 1959 for some stiffness and aching on the top of her shoulders. A second course of bee venom was started, the last treatment being on April 23, 1959, at which time she had received her third complete plaque. She had at this time about 90% recovery, was much more comfortable and has had no reason to return. My last contact with this patient was by telephone November 16, 1961 at which time she stated that she had had no recurrence of her trouble and was able to do everything.

Mr. S. K., age 38, acute polyarthritis. First seen March 14, 1957 with acute inflammatory changes in ankles, knees, hands of about two years' duration. He appeared at the office at this time on crutches, having imbibed of alcoholic beverages rather heavily during preceding few weeks to relieve pain. He was given analgesics, told to stop drinking because of the effect alcohol has in impairing successful bee venom therapy. He was seen again April 14, 1957 and was started on bee venom every other day until the first of June, at which time he had had four complete plaques and was moderately improved. He was seen on July 8, 1957 for a slight flareup and was given one treatment with bee venom. He has been able to resume his regular work following the final treatment and when last seen March 4, 1960 had had no further recurrance and was able to do a full day's work.

Mrs. D. C., age 31, rheumatoid arthritis and rheumatic heart disease. This mother of five children was seen on December 29, 1959 for pain, swelling of her fingers, bilateral metacarpal phalangeal joints, both knees, both hips, complaining of morning stiffness of several months' duration. Latex fixation was positive. She was started on bee venom tablets on February 6, 1960, taking one tablet every other day until 23 tablets had been taken. This course of treatment resulted in moderate improvement in all joints. In May, 1957 she appeared again with recurrence of pains which were aggravated caring for all of her children and livestock. She was started May, 1961 on a second course of Buccal bee venom tablets which were continued through July 25, 1961 at which time she felt much better and had maintained her improvement for one month with marked improvement in her grip. Because of the presence of symptoms she was started on a third course of bee venom tablets in September, 1961, finishing the last of these about the middle of November. All her joints were much better but tended to be aggravated by heavy work such as carrying pails of water. She is still under treatment but has made very satisfactory progress.

Very truly yours,
HERMANN N. SANDER, M.D.

APPENDIX J

Adverse Reports and Their Critiques

Dr. F. B. Paddock, apiarist of the state of Iowa, wrote a pamphlet in 1952 on the subject of bee venom. He reviewed the literature. We reprint part of his review here:

(USE OF BEE VENOM IN MEDICINE)

The most thorough review of the use of bee venom in medicine up to 1935 was presented by Bodog F. Beck in his well known book "Bee Venom Therapy." In the present article, the medicinal use of bee venom will be reviewed from papers published since 1935. Cases reported in non-medical or popular literature will not be included.

In his discourse on bee venom therapy in chronic rheumatic disorders Burt [Dr. J. B. Burt of England] states: "Few things are more difficult to assess than the value of a special therapeutic agent in treatment of a chronic disease like rheumatoid arthritis and chronic rheumatism, unless, of course, the remedy is specific: and bee venom is by no means a specific cure. In rheumatoid arthritis there is an even larger psychological factor than in most chronic diseases. A method of treatment such as bee venom, which has a popular reputation emphasized by laymen for commercial purposes, undoubtedly appeals to the imagination. But taking everything into consideration, the writer is of the opinion that bee venom is of definite value in certain cases of chronic rheumatism."

Many physicians have experimented with injectable bee venom and have published reports. The results of the treatment appear to have been extremely variable. According to Burt, bee venom is chiefly of value in the treatment of fibrositis, particularly where the nodules in the muscles or fascia do not clear up by simple physical treatment. It has been strongly advocated for the treatment of sciatic and brachial neuritis and bee venom is useful where the case is due to fibrositis of structures in relation to the nerves. Cases of sciatic and brachial neuritis due to other causes, such as osteoarthritis of the vertebral joints, do not appear to respond to this treatment.

In rheumatoid arthritis good results have been obtained, particularly in men, where the disease is under two years duration. Burt has treated something like 200 cases of typical rheumatoid arthritis showing rapid sedimentation rate and osteoporosis with bee venom. In no case were there any bad results such as may be produced by treatment with vaccines or gold, and in a few cases the results were really good. Burt has been surprised by the number of persons who on returning to the hospital, asked for a repetition of this treatment and who assigned their previous improvement to bee venom. About eight hours after injection all cases which appeared to benefit showed some general reaction, such as slight swelling of the joints or generalized aches. This happened so often that it was not Burt's custom to continue treatment, unless there was a slight general reaction.

The above is from the *British Journal of Physical Medicine,* 1939. It is "Bee Venom Therapy in Chronic Rheumatic Disorders" by the previously mentioned Dr. Burt:

Nichols (1938) of Cornell University Medical College treated 27 patients with severe active rheumatoid arthritis with the stings of the honey bees. Five had to discontinue the treatment after a few weeks because of severe local or general reactions. Two stopped because they found the treatment disagreeable. Twenty continued the bee stings for from three to 18 months and received from 53 to 1,434 stings. Three of the patients were markedly improved, five remained the same, seven became very much worse. Nichols concluded: "Bee sting therapy had no constant or noteworthy effects in treatment of rheumatoid arthritis. The results were so discouraging that we felt we were not justified in continuing this form of treatment."

The above report by Dr. Nichols is discussed in detail by Dr. B. F. Beck, in a letter he wrote to Dr. Nichols on November 23, 1938, which is reprinted in full in this Appendix.

From the *American Journal of the Medical Sciences,* June, 1941, we report on an article on Bee Venom by J. L. Hollander of the U.S.A.:

Hollander (1941), at the Pennsylvania Hospital in Philadelphia, in a controlled experiment used 59 patients suffering from rheumatic diseases (38 females and 21 males, with ages ranging from 23 to 69 years and the duration of the disease from five months to 33 years). Only the injection of bee venom in solution was given during the period of observation. Forty-two patients were treated with bee venom solution and 17, serving as controls, were given non-specific solution. (Remark of the editor of the journal in which the paper was published: "The word 'control' must be accepted with reservation, as 'control' would, strictly speaking, require the use of a therapeutically inert material, not one that produces non-specific protein shock. It must be kept in mind that non-specific protein reaction may at times be helpful in arthritis and that the effect of bee stings themselves may be a part of such a non-specific protein reaction.") The dosage was increased twice a week until the patient received the equivalent of 10 to 30 bee stings per visit. Only patients treated more than six times were included in the series. Most of the patients received 20 or more injections or received the equivalent of more than 100 bee stings. Each of the patients in the control group were given 15 injections of a milk-protein solution, intra-muscularly or intra-venously, at weekly intervals. None of the 42 patients with chronic arthritis who were treated with bee venom solution was completely relieved of his disease. Three patients were greatly improved, five were moderately but perceptively better and nine experienced some relief during the course of treatment but relapsed soon after the injections were discontinued. Twenty-two patients were unaffected by the bee venom therapy, and three were definitely worse after treatment. In the controls three were moderately improved, five were better while receiving injections but they obtained no lasting benefits. Nine were unchanged. There were no ill effects.

The length of treatment and actual number of injections did not have direct effect on the degree of improvement. In the patients showing lasting benefits from the venom treatment the average number of visits was 18, with improvement showing itself as early as the third visit. In the unimproved group the average number of treatments was 21, with one patient experiencing no change after 32 injections. The patients made worse by the treatment had eight, nine and 17 injections respectively.

The most marked improvement following bee venom therapy was seen in the case of fibrositis, in which an almost complete remission of symptoms occurred. Reichart and other workers have found that fibrositis is more responsive than rheumatoid arthritis. One case of advanced and one case of early atrophic arthritis showed great improvement.

The most interesting, and perhaps most significant case, was that of J.R. For 23 years this man had suffered from rheumatoid arthritis, and his principal occupation for the past 18 years was keeping bees! He had been stung hundreds of times and he had "sold" bee stings to other arthritics but still had the complaints and deformities characteristic of advanced atrophic arthritis. This patient was given a course of bee venom injections with no improvements at all.

Hollander concluded: "The incidence and degree of improvement were very discouraging, and all but one of the patients (the one suffering from fibrositis) are still seeking relief from their disease. Even though a few patients showed definite and lasting improvements, it is felt that a painful, tedious, expensive and somewhat toxic form of therapy should yield much better results to justify its continued use."

The author offers a detailed discussion of Dr. Hollander's entire report, of which the above is only a part, in order to show how errors either in the selection of cases, in the technique employed or in the conclusions reached can be made misleading. The facts cited here apply in all instances in which poor or outmoded technique has been used. They can, therefore, serve as an outstanding example. Dr. Hollander is still in practice and can reply if he wishes; his report was selected for discussion in preference to that of another author, who might be deceased.

Referring to the work of Kroner and coworkers, Hollander mentions that "they reported no cures, but 35 patients were markedly improved by the treatment." In another portion of his report, Hollander quotes Kroner that "relief from pain was reported to be definite and lasting."

An open-minded investigator would know that "cures" could not ethically have been claimed without waiting two to three years longer to make certain that the improvements were permanent. Had Kroner claimed "cures" so soon, when the report was written, he would have merited just criticism.

Hollander refers to the unfavorable report by Dr. Nichols, who was on Kroner's team, which rendered a favorable report.

It is well known by those experienced with the bee venom therapy (Schick) that the natural secretion of the honey bee as it is deposited into the circulation of the human body during a bee sting is best in quality and that no injectable product of bee venom can be as good or better. How and why Nichols came to the contrary conclusion may be explained by the letter written by the late Dr. Bodog F. Beck to Nichols, published in this Appendix.

Hollander took (not selected) the patients for his "study" at random. He gives no X-ray findings, sedimentation rates or other information which would give some idea of the stages of the arthritic cases. Those with severe joint changes—with complete or nearly complete destruction and obliteration of the joints—naturally would not respond favorably. Neither present methods, nor any to be developed in future, can be expected to overcome such unfortunate conditions. Only transplantation, if this is ever mastered, might do it, but even this is extremely doubtful. Let us remember that Hollander reports some of his cases had been afflicted for up to 33 years; and he was evidently in a hurry for results. One needs to be reasonable in such matters. Patients react differently to bee venom and the physician using this therapy must know how to interpret normal developments.

As for "controls" used by Hollander in his study, Paddock has already dealt with that subject in his own report from the literature.

"The number of bee stings," says Hollander, "given to patients were increased until the patient received the equivalent of 10 to 30 bee stings per visit. The amount given was determined by the individual reaction to the solution."

It is absurd to expect "cures" or even improvement in chronic arthritic cases with such low dosages. Normal local reactions during treatment are favorable signs and they are usually welcome as such, because they indicate good results soon to follow. Hollander evidently did not know this, so he discontinued the treatments. This author tells each patient in advance about such reactions, so they welcome them when they come instead of being temporarily discouraged by them. Patients under bee venom therapy do not usually show any signs of improvement until those normal, local reactions develop.

"Only patients treated more than six times were included in this series," reports Hollander. "Most of the patients were injected twenty times or more, or received the equivalent of more than 100 bee stings."

With such technique one can wonder that any improvements were shown at all. The Kroner team of five physicians report using up to 52 injections and they kept their patients under treatment for from one to 14 months, which Hollander did not do; he continued the treatment only up to ten weeks.

It is important to note the statement by Hollander that "no untoward reactions occurred in these cases." That being so, why does he state in his "conclusions" that the bee venom method "is somewhat toxic"? As a matter of fact, no other investigator who knew the proper technique has found it toxic.

Modern knowledge teaches that we should not judge empirically the length of treatment with bee venom or the number of injections to be given any patient. It should be done with more precision. Close observation of the wheals as they first develop, their size, roundness and regularity, compared with their later size, irregularity, serrated and edematous appearance, gives us the needed scientific information. As the treatment continues, the individual wheals outstretch toward the neighboring wheals until they fuse and, finally, form one large wheal. When this fusion is complete, it is proof that the patient has become saturated and that only three or four more injections are needed and that particular series of injections is over. Nothing useful can be accomplished unless the patient has been saturated; that result is the very essence of the treatment.

These scientific indications and developments are neither mentioned nor used by Hollander. Did he know them?

Furthermore, modern technique has taught us that after the patient has become saturated, he or she is given a vacation from treatment lasting from three to six weeks, depending upon the nature of the rheumatic condition. After this an evaluation of the case is made and a decision is reached as to whether further treatment is indicated. Very chronic cases need several such series. On this phase of the subject, Hollander states simply: "In several instances the local reaction was excessive, the wheals showing pseudopod formation, and edema of the area ensued."

It does seem that the normal scientific developments were not understood.

Hollander quotes only from unfavorable sources whose poor results were perhaps due to similar lack of knowledge of the proper technique to be employed. The many hundreds of good results reported from numerous university centers abroad, including Russia, where much of this work has already been done, are either not mentioned at all or else the details are entirely withheld.

Even when he reports a good result among his own patients, he does it reluctantly, as:

> One case of advanced atrophic arthritis showed a definite symptomatic and objective improvement. This woman had been very much discouraged with results from other forms of treatment but improved definitely with the use of bee venom. Pain, swelling, and stiffness of the diseased joints was decreased, her mental health became better, and the blood count and sedimentation rate improved. *The good results in the early case of rheumatoid arthritis must be at least partially credited to the removal of diseased tonsils 6 weeks before treatment began.* (underlined by author)

Finally, Hollander states:

> The most interesting, and perhaps the most significant, case was that of J.R. For 23 years this man had suffered from rheumatoid arthritis, and his principal occupation for the past 18 years was keeping bees. He had been stung hundreds of times and he had "sold" bee stings to other arthritics, but still had the complaints and deformities characteristic of advanced atrophic arthritis. This patient was given a course of bee venom injections with no improvement at all. It must be stated, however, that he was actually immune

to bee stings, there being no local or general reaction following large doses of venom.

A case like the above is simple to understand and to explain by one experienced with the therapy. The immunity is due to the fact that the patient became *saturated* with the venom. Furthermore, if the early stages of the arthritis resulted in severe joint changes—irreversible changes—before he became a beekeeper, or even after he became a beekeeper but before he received adequate doses of the venom at proper intervals, as seems the case here, no results—or very little—could be expected for reasons already given.

In addition, having been "stung hundreds of times" is not in itself necessarily helpful.

To get results, the administration of the venom should be systematic, persistent, in constantly but gradually increased quantities and under scientific supervision. It is true that cases have been reported of a person suffering from arthritis and being overwhelmed by angry swarms of bees who stung him mercilessly hundreds of times and the sufferer was soon cured of his arthritis. Some such sufferers may also have died as a result. Scientific medicine does not recommend such risky and doubtful medical care from physicians.

Finally, the conclusions reached by Hollander are erroneous, since they are based on easily avoidable errors in technique and apparent lack of knowledge of the general subject under consideration.

Cohen and coworkers, U.S.A., "Bee Venom in the Treatment of Chronic Arthritis," *Pennsylvania Medical Journal,* 1942:

In discussing their treatment of rheumatic diseases with bee venom, Cohen and coworkers (1942) stated in the introduction to their paper: "In the mind of many physicians the bee venom has had associated with it the stigma of charlatanism. This concept has undoubtedly grown from the fact that many of the reports have been unscientific and the claims made for bee venom have often been too extravagant. The present authors felt that a critical trial of this therapeutic agent was in order." They tried to evaluate bee venom as a therapeutic agent in treatment of arthritis regardless of type. Magnesium sulfate (12.5 per cent) and glucose (10 per cent) were used as controls. Both these substances were selected because they are similar to bee venom only in that they act as irritants and cause a stinging sensation when injected intradermally.

The authors found that bee venom is a good therapeutic agent in treatment of pain in arthritis regardless of type. They were inclined to believe that bee venom acts as a counterirritant, producing capillary engorgement at the site of treatment. Magnesium sulfate and glucose gave results comparable to those of bee venom. No appreciable change in the sedimentation rate could be elicited. Use of bee venom, however, showed marked improvement in considerably fewer cases than did the use of either magnesium sulfate or glucose.

F. S. McKenna, Medical Press, 1949:

[McKenna] (1939) successfully treated some mild cases of rheumatism with Forapin injections.

"Of twenty-two patients (eight males and 14 females, ages 26-83) which Montgomery (1940) treated with injectable bee venom (Sharp and Dohme 'Lyovec') 11 showed a marked improvement, nine were considerably improved and two did not show any improvement. (One had neuritis associated with pregnancy and the other patient fell and injured her back and could not continue the treatment.)"

Bayne, *Southern Surgeon,* March, 1948:

[Bayne] (1948) treated seven attacks of tic douloureux (spasmodic facial neuralgia) in five patients with bee venom with excellent results. The pain was greatly diminished in all cases in 45 minutes to one hour. The bee venom relieved pain which was not relieved by a half grain of morphine. The venom was given intradermally at the site of pain. The pain, if it recurred, came gradually and the patient had time to get back for treatment before it was very severe. The average length of the treatment was two to three weeks and, in most instances, the last injection was given after a week without pain. Bee venom caused an immediate hyperemia in the area involved and apparently had an effect which lasted from 12 to 24 hours.

F.E. Guyton, U.S.A., "Bee Sting Therapy for Arthritis and Neuritis," *Journal Econ. Entom.*, 1947:

[Guyton] (1947) used bee stings in treatment of varying arthritic conditions. Before treatment began, each patient was required to have a thorough examination by the family physician or a specialist, and the physician was asked to make a request for the treatment. The first treatment consisted of a test sting in order to show the patient's reaction. Regular treatment was begun if there were no unusual reactions to the test sting. The stings were placed on the affected area and allowed to remain imbedded for three to five minutes. The bees were handled with forceps and the stings were removed with forceps. Applications of stings were made at intervals of three to four days.

Guyton treated six patients with bee stings for arthritis and neuritis. One patient was treated for three different occurrences of arthritis. Another patient was treated for two different occurrences in the same area. A year intervened between the first and the second occurrence. Three of the six cases treated experienced complete recovery with the application of from two to 16 stings. A ten-year chronic case with acute flareups was given 502 stings over a period of one year. There was great benefit from the treatment but no cure. All cases treated showed improved conditions. Three cases out of six became supersensitive to bee stings. In one case a check was run. It was agreed with the patient to treat only the most swollen knee and finger, leaving the other knee and fingers as checks. After about a month's treatment, the treated knee became almost normal. The other knee remained unchanged. The patient asked that treatment should be extended to the untreated knee. Because of the developed sensitiveness the treatment was discontinued.

The following are comments by F.B. Paddock, apiarist of the state of Iowa, following his study of the medical literature:

From the foregoing review of literature it is clearly evident that in many cases bee venom treatment brought a marked improvement or a complete cure to sufferers from rheumatic diseases. Even in the series where the general results were negative, there was a certain number of individuals who were benefited. In using bee venom as a treatment for rheumatic disorders one has to bear in mind that in some chronic cases, as Tertsch pointed out, there is no sign of improvement until the patient begins to react to bee stings. This reaction is important (see Burt's observation) and it may appear sometimes after as many as a thousand bee stings have been applied. In treating some obstinate cases of arthritis Tertsch used as many as 15,000 stings to achieve the cure. Moreover, the same individual may, at different times, react to the bee sting in different ways, depending on his physiological condition. It should also be pointed out that the negative conclusion reported in some of the papers reviewed were drawn after the application of the relatively small number of bee stings, or their equivalent in solution (Nichols from 53 to 1,434; Hollander more than 100 bee stings). Apparently more controlled experiments are desirable to bring the final answer to this controversial question.

CAUTION: What must not be overlooked is the fact that nearly all clinical and research reports in this volume date back several years, some a great many years.

Recent research work here and in other countries together with improvement in technique assure far better results than were obtained in earlier periods.

APPENDIX K

A Short Note on Bee Venom Therapy In South America

by EDUARDO MARTINEZ RUBIO
(Tucumán, Argentina)

Bee venom treatment was intensively initiated in 1936, when E. Martinez Rubio discovered a crystallization technique which made the toxin better tolerable and painless. The product is available under the brand name APITOXINA, and Drs. F. Rawak and Mussio Furnier have established a clinic for apitherapy in Montevideo where they have treated up to this date more than 5,000 patients with various rheumatic and arthritic conditions.

In Argentina, Dr. Barcelo Torrents and Dr. Alberto Torino, Buenos Aires, widely initiated clinical treatment with PERPHYSIN, an injectable preparation prepared from the Apitoxin of Dr. Rubio. Up to the present date, these physicians have treated more than 8,000 patients with various rheumatic conditions.

Since the foundation of the *Instituto Biogenetico Rubio* in Tucumán (Argentina), an ever increasing number of physicians employ this therapy with success and enthusiasm due to the potent curative action and limited toxicity of APITOXINA. More than 60,000 ampoules have been sent out by this modern institution with 5,000 bee colonies for obtaining the necessary raw material. It is exported to various countries.

In the Laboratories APITROP, ampoules and ointments on the basis of bee venom (apitoxina) are prepared. This product is the most widely used in Argentina in the rheumatic field.

INDEX

INDEX

Made in the USA
Monee, IL
04 November 2026

67387177R00125